Global Oncology

Harvard Global Health Catalyst summit lecture notes

Global Oncology

Harvard Global Health Catalyst summit lecture notes

Wilfred Ngwa
Harvard University and University of Massachusetts

Paul Nguyen
Harvard University

IOP Publishing, Bristol, UK

ISBN 978-0-7503-1359-9 (ebook)
ISBN 978-0-7503-1360-5 (print)
ISBN 978-03-750-1361-2 (mobi)

DOI 10.1088/978-0-7503-1359-9

Version: 20170801

IOP Expanding Physics
ISSN 2053-2563 (online)
ISSN 2054-7315 (print)

British Library Cataloguing-in-Publication Data: A catalogue record for this book is available from the British Library.

Published by IOP Publishing, wholly owned by The Institute of Physics, London

IOP Publishing, Temple Circus, Temple Way, Bristol, BS1 6HG, UK

US Office: IOP Publishing, Inc., 190 North Independence Mall West, Suite 601, Philadelphia, PA 19106, USA

We have a dream that one day cancer will be eradicated and that people of all socioeconomic, racial, religious and cultural backgrounds will have access to quality treatment. We dedicate this book to anyone dealing with cancer, and especially to those in low and middle-income countries in Asia, Africa, Latin America, eastern Europe and elsewhere who have little or no access to cancer treatment and radiotherapy

Contents

Foreword

International collaboration on cancer-related issues is one of the main global scientific activities at the moment. This is also emphasized in the recent WHO Report 'Cancer prevention and control in the context of an integrated approach' [1] and the related statement of the International Union for Cancer Care (IUCC), supported by the IOMP.

The activities described in this book, part of the Global Health Catalyst (GHC) Summit at Harvard, describe exactly such an integrated approach—which is vital for low and middle-income countries (LMICs). Without doubt the activities of the Summit and the expertise, shared in the book, will have high international impact and will trigger further collaborations in the field.

The subject of the book is very much in line with the work of medical physicists, united under the International Organization for Medical Physics (IOMP) [2]. This is stated in the IOMP mission 'to advance medical physics practice worldwide by disseminating scientific and technical information, fostering the educational and professional development of medical physics and promoting the highest quality medical services for patients'. The majority of medical physicists work in the field of radiotherapy and their work is directly related to cancer diagnosis and treatment. One of the priorities of IOMP is in line with the topics in the current book—help for our colleagues in LMICs and Africa in particular [3]. The need for specific training courses and increase of human resources in this field are more than obvious. Currently in Africa there are working fewer than 500 medical physicists (about 2% of all medical physicists in the world), most them in the field of radiotherapy. This small number of medical physicists does not correlate with the fact that about 15% of the people on the planet live in Africa, and underlines the need for active steps, as discussed in the current book.

The book includes the proceedings from the 2016 GHC Summit. It outlines unique approaches, supported by the success of the Harvard GHC, which has gathered huge support from various parties—from the realms of politics, professional bodies, industry and most importantly—the LMICs diaspora. The structure of the book reflects this multi-faceted line of development—ranging from education and research to industry perspective and views of various society members. The book comes just in time to be seen in parallel with the recently published 'WHO list of priority medical devices for cancer management' [4].

The chapter on education is very important, it emphasizes the use of e-learning and knowledge sharing —vital elements of the process in LMICs. The chapter gathers the experience of key-players in the field: The American Society for Radiation Oncology (ASTRO); The African Organization for Research and Training in Cancer (AORTIC); The American Association for Physicists in Medicine (AAPM); The Federation of African Medical Physics Organization (FAMPO) and other global oncology education initiatives (both AAPM and FAMPO are members of IOMP). Medical physics is one of the world leaders in the field of e-learning and it is only natural that the profession supports the goals of the present book. Special acknowledgement is due to the firm support of AAPM for colleagues from LMICs, for example by making available to them the Virtual Library of AAPM.

I could add to the above e-learning resources the free online *Encyclopaedia of Medical Physics* plus *Multilingual Dictionary of Terms* (in 29 languages) [5]—this reference material includes many topics which can be useful for the education in radiotherapy medical physics.

Last year IOMP published in its e-Journal *Medical Physics International* (www.mpijournal.org) a review of the excellent e-book of W Ngwa and T Ngoma *Emerging Models for Radiation Oncology Global Health* [6].

The current book *Global Oncology: Harvard Global Health Catalyst summit lecture notes*, edited by Wilfred Ngwa and Paul Nguyen, is another important step in the direction of support for LMICs and IOMP will further disseminate it to its members.

Slavik Tabakov PhD, Dr h.c.
(President International Organization for Medical Physics, IOMP)

References

[1] WHO Executive Board 140th session 2017 Cancer prevention and control in the context of an integrated approach, EB140/31

[2] International Organization for Medical Physics www.iomp.org

[3] Tabakov S 2014 IOMP Project supporting the development of medical physics in Africa in collaboration with IAEA and WHO *J. Med. Phys. Int.* http://mpijournal.org/MPI-v02i01.aspx

[4] World Health Organization 2017 *WHO List of Priority Medical Devices for Cancer Management* http://www.who.int/medical_devices/publications/priority_med_dev_cancer_management/en/

[5] EMITEL Encyclopaedia of medical Physics plus Multilingual Dictionary of Terms www.emitel2.eu

[6] Ngwa W and Ngoma T 2016 *Emerging Models for Radiation Oncology Global Health* (Bristol: IOP Publishing)

Foreword

It is beautiful to see 'Harambee' in action. All are pulling together, for a common goal and a sense of community. The participants in the 2016 Global Health Catalyst Summit represented a broad spectrum of languages and perspectives and personalities and talents, but they shared the same lofty aspiration, so well stated in the event's vision statement:

> *We have a dream that one day, cancer will be eradicated, and that people of all socio-economic, racial, religious, and cultural backgrounds will have access to quality healthcare.*

Turning that dream into a reality will require lots of *harambee*, but there is a reason to be hopeful. It should be appreciated, first of all, that as recently as perhaps twenty or thirty years ago, an intensive focus on screening and treatment of malignancies in developing countries would have been misplaced energy, since for so long the major public health challenges were in the realm of infectious diseases and other non-cancerous conditions. However, according to the Global Burden of Disease Study of 2010, the number of deaths due to communicable, maternal, neonatal, and nutritional disorders dropped worldwide by 17% over the prior 20 years [1]. It was thanks to the massive collaborative efforts of governments, private companies, philanthropic organizations and local community groups working step by step for many years to surmount the environmental, political and educational hurdles required to put such an enormous dent in the annual death tolls of these largely preventable conditions. Of course, this laudable progress has not unexpectedly redefined the major healthcare challenges in many areas, as deaths due to neoplasm rose by 38% over that same period [1].

To suggest that those of us fortunate enough to live in wealthy countries with easy access to high quality medical care across the board, and excellent cancer care in particular, have an ethical and moral duty to lend a hand to those in less privileged regions is a statement of the obvious, but it might not convey the best reasons why we should have a generous spirit in this regard. At least equally compelling, in my view, is that there is so much to learn and so much to enjoy from the personal relationships that can grow when innovators from many sectors in many countries all pull together.

I hope that these lecture notes will give readers a sense of the *harambee* that was felt at the meeting, and I hope that the collaborations and knowledge exchanges that happen as a result of the Global Health Catalyst Summit meetings propel us all forward so that the Global Burden of Disease Study of 2030 will show the same progress in reducing mortality from malignant disease that we have seen in other forms of illness.

Brian D Kavanagh, MD, MPH
University of Colorado
President, American Society for Radiation Oncology

Reference

[1] Lozano R, Naghavi M and Foreman K *et al* 2013 Global and regional mortality from 235 causes of death for 20 age groups in 1990 and 2010: a systematic analysis for the global burden of disease study 2010 *The Lancet* **380** 2095–128

Preface

As the stark inequality in cancer access and outcomes across the globe gradually enters the consciousness of the intellectual and international community, global oncology emerges as a sphere of actions and interventions to close this divide. Many young oncologists in both High Income Countries (HICs) and Low and Middle Income Countries (LMICs) have shown a growing interest in global oncology as a career path [1,2]. Mine was spurred by my experiences in cancer care, both as a medical student and as a young medical practitioner in southern Nigeria. I remember working with healthcare providers with little to no oncology training, making up for the deficit of trained oncologists. Our referred patients had to travel a long distance to receive a course of radiotherapy, surgery, chemotherapy or radiologic evaluations. Treatment default was not uncommon. I witnessed many families go into bankruptcy, and some children temporarily drop out of school so the family could afford treatment for a close relative with a diagnosis of cancer [3]. These clinical experiences molded my aspiration for leadership in the policy, economics, research, education, and clinical aspect of cancer care in low and middle-income countries. And it was in the pursuit of further leadership and experiential training that I realized the domain of global health training for future oncology leaders was yet to be defined [2].

The consolidation of global oncology as a sub-specialization necessitates a coordinated cross-pollination of ideas between a range of experts in global oncology care. These include healthcare providers, advocates, policy-makers, business leaders, global health economists, academicians and other health personnel at all levels who utilize or implement healthcare services for underserved populations. Moreover, the development of a sustainable capacity and infrastructure for clinical oncology care, research, and education in LMICs will require partnership with the oncology community of high-income countries. The emerging global oncology sphere is currently dynamic with a yet-to-be-defined rigid curriculum, and a platform is necessary for this partnership as well as an up-to-date dissemination of information, perspectives and sharing of oncology initiatives in LMICs. The Global Health Catalyst (GHC) summits at Harvard Medical School fulfill this demand. It is thus, at the recommendation of academicians, oncologists and global health practitioners from around the globe, that the GHC has begun the publication of lecture notes at its annual summit. These notes, based on information shared by world experts at the 2016 summit, will help educate future leaders and anyone interested in global health on the issues of global oncology from its core principles, to cancer burden, and to an understanding of the ongoing and emerging initiatives. With a broad range of conference speakers, this text has an interdisciplinary tone, mixing approaches and perspectives to describe and analyze solutions for oncology services in global health efforts. Its scope covers global oncology education, research, care, and outreaches, with a chapter on frequently asked questions in global oncology and a final chapter that discusses the global oncology moonshot and other emerging initiatives and innovations in the burgeoning field of global oncology.

Omoruyi Credit Irabor MD MPH
Global Health Catalyst
Harvard Medical School

References

[1] Ngwa W and Ngoma T 2016 *Emerging Models for Global Health in Radiation Oncology* (Bristol: IOP Publishing)
[2] Grover S, Balogun O D and Yamoah K *et al* 2015 Training global oncologists: addressing the global cancer control problem *Front. Oncol.* **5** 80
[3] Irabor O C, Nwankwo K C and Adewuyi S A 2016 The stagnation and decay of radiation oncology resources: lessons from nigeria *Int. J. Radiat. Oncol. Biol. Phys.* **95** 1327–33

Acknowledgements

We acknowledge support from many who have helped in organizing, moderating, and chairing different sessions of the Global Health Catalyst summits at Harvard Medical School. Special acknowledgement and thanks are due to:

Mike Makrigiorgos, PhD (Dana Farber/Harvard Cancer Center)
Daphne Haas-Kogan, MD (Dana Farber/Harvard Cancer Center)
Erno Sajo, PhD (University of Massachusetts, Lowell)
Matthew Katz, MD (Radiation Nation)
Twalib Ngoma, MD (MUHAS Tanzania)
Akila Viswanathan, MD (John Hopkins University)
Ahmed Elzawawy, MD (AORTIC, ICEDOC)
Ernest Okonkwo (Mephida, Germany)
Folakemi Odedina, PhD (University of Florida, AORTIC)
Thomas Randall, MD (Dana Farber/Harvard Cancer Center)
Stephen Avery, PhD (University of Pennsylvania School of Medicine)
Onyinye Balogun, MD (Weill Cornell Medical College)
Makeda Williams, PhD (NIH)
Julie Pollard, PhD (MD Anderson Cancer Center)
Lydia Asana (African Renaissance Ambassador Corp, USA)
Kwanele Asante (AORTIC)
Christian Ntizimira, MD (Rwanda)
Thomas Winningham, PhD (Health First, ARA)
Sulma Mohammed, PhD (Purdue University, AORTIC)
Kenneth Numfor, PhD (ARA)
Victor Mbarika, PhD (ICT University)
Elizabeth Omondi (Cancer Africa)
Hariet Shangarai, RN (NesiWangu.com, Washington DC)
Emmanuel Ngassa, MD (Ask Docta, Germany/Cameroon)
Doyin Oluwole, MD (Global Health Innovations and Action Foundation)
Oscar Nebangwa, MBA (ARA Corp)
Nazik Hammad, MD (AORTIC)
Stella Adamu (Patcha Foundation)

The Global Health Catalyst summits received seed-funding from Dana Farber Cancer Institute, Brigham and Women's Hospital, and the Radcliffe Institute for Advanced Studies at Harvard University. Additional yearly sponsors for this important global health event are also acknowledged.

Author biographies

Wilfred Ngwa

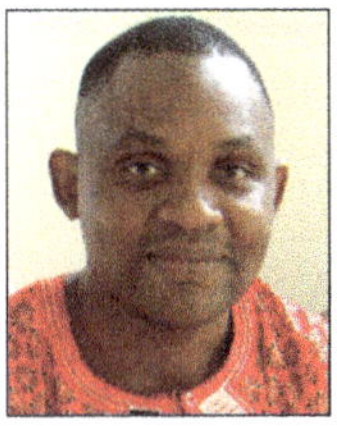

Wilfred Ngwa, PhD, is the Director of the Global Health Catalyst program at Dana–Farber/Harvard Cancer Center and a professor of radiation oncology and faculty medical physicist at Harvard Medical School and the University of Massachusetts. He also currently holds an international guest professorship at the University of Heidelberg, Germany. He has published a number of books including a previous book on global health: *Emerging Models for Global Health in Radiation Oncology*. He has won a number of awards and prizes, including the 2015 BRIght Futures Prize for innovative new technology designed for use during radiotherapy to kill cancer cells that have spread to other parts of the body.

Paul L Nguyen

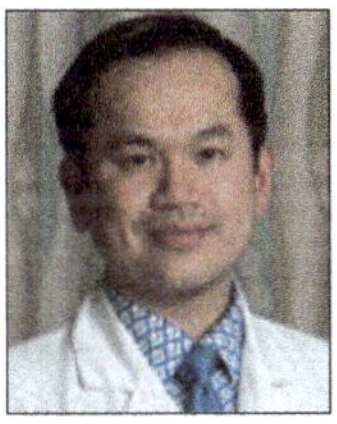

Paul L Nguyen, MD, is Associate Professor of Radiation Oncology at Harvard Medical School and Vice-Chair for Clinical Research in the Department of Radiation Oncology, Dana–Farber Cancer Institute, Brigham and Women's Hospital. Over the last years, he has helped chair and co-direct the yearly Global Health Catalyst summits at Harvard Medical School. He has been a recipient of many awards, including the Harvard College Award for Excellence in Teaching and Harvard Medical School Teaching awards. He is chair-elect of the ASCO/ASTRO/SUO Genitourinary Cancers Symposium and senior Associate Editor of the *International Journal of Radiation Oncology, Biology, and Physics*.

Chapter 1

Introduction

1.1 Global oncology and the Harvard Global Health Catalyst summits

In November 2012, the then Director of the National Cancer Institute and leaders in cancer research and policy from 15 economically diverse countries met at the US National Institutes of Health to discuss opportunities to reduce cancer incidence and mortality, improve cancer care, and increase our understanding of disease pathophysiology. The emerging consensus from the meeting was that successful campaigns to control cancer will increasingly depend on concerted international collaborations [1]. The recent World Health Organization Cancer Report highlights the urgency for such international collaborations, with over 60% of 14 million new cancer cases and 70% of 8.2 million deaths per year occurring in low and middle income countries (LMICs), some of which, sadly, are the least capable of dealing with cancer without some form of collaboration.

Interestingly, there has been a recent major upsurge of interest in global health amongst oncology health professionals. Unfortunately, significant barriers remain in initiating or participating in international collaborations in global oncology. These barriers include: geographic or space/time, systematic, and cultural barriers [2–4]. Addressing these barriers to collaboration is crucial, given the rising global burden of cancer, and other non-communicable diseases.

The Harvard Global Health Catalyst (GHC) (figure 1.1) is designed to catalyze high impact international collaborations, providing a solution to overcome the geographic, systematic, and cultural barriers to global health collaborations. To address the geographic or space/time barrier, the GHC organizes yearly summits which bring together stakeholders from high income countries (HICs) and LMICs to share knowledge, network, and collaborate. The objective is to seed new collaborations or strengthen existing ones. The GHC approach is modeled after the successful collaboration-driven model of Harvard Catalyst, which fosters a culture of collaboration in 31 Harvard-affiliated institutions, hospitals, and community

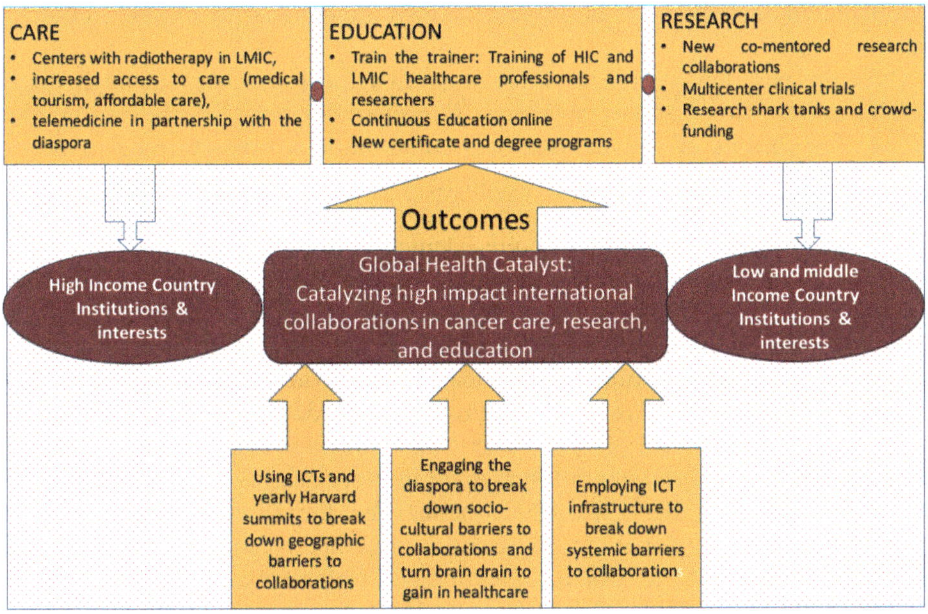

Figure 1.1. Harvard Global Health Catalyst model for catalyzing high impact international collaborations to address the growing global burden of cancer. ICT = information and communication technologies; HIC = high income countries; LMIC = Low and Middle Income Countries.

partners. The GHC is an extension of this model to include a growing number of institutions, each year, from HICs and LMICs. Beyond the face-to-face GHC summits, an information and communications technology (ICT) platform is being developed to provide a systematic way for investigators from HIC and LMIC institutions to easily find each other and form teams, share tools and technologies, receive advanced research education/training, obtain seed funding for collaborative or co-mentored research involving HICs and HIC faculty, which can lead to joint publications and major subsequent additional joint funding.

A unique approach of the Harvard GHC is its unprecedented level of engagement with government leaders, industry, advocates, and community organizations such as diaspora organizations. Outreach involvement of diasporas in collaborations is expected to help minimize cultural barriers, given the diasporas' better appreciation of both HICs and the sending LMIC cultures. In addition to catalyzing stronger culturally sensitive collaborations, the participation of the diasporas can help turn the brain drain into a gain against cancer. The diasporas' passion for contributing to their sending countries, and substantial human resource and financial potential (e.g. over $50 billion per year in remittances by the African diaspora) is a significant asset, including in supporting crowdfunding, and cancer prevention awareness/education and advocacy. Also, the involvement of industry in the GHC summits is significant in facilitating transfer of new knowledge to practical healthcare solutions, economic growth, and sustainable development. Involvement of government leaders—ministers of health and ambassadors—is designed to help drive policy to address cancer in a sustainable way.

Over the past few years, the GHC summit's focus has been on high impact collaborations with LMICs in Africa. Expected outcomes at the yearly event include: the seeding of new international collaborations; strengthening of existing collaborations to reduce global health disparities; global oncology online courses; co-mentored diaspora-funded research microgrants; telemedicine and virtual medical missions; award recognition; unprecedented partnerships with sports, religion, industry, and diasporas, to address global health disparities; ICT-powered care research and education programs; knowledge sharing; and publications for disseminating the new knowledge from the summit.

During the yearly summit, global health leaders and key stakeholders share cutting-edge knowledge, through the means of highly educational lectures, which are shaping the emerging field of global oncology. This book is a compilation of some lectures/talks given at the summit, presented in more detail.

Unique features of this book include the fact that the material presented is really at the cutting-edge of global oncology, and is presented by some of the best leaders and key-stakeholders. The book includes highly illuminative examples and addresses the frequently asked questions in global oncology, documented from the summit. It can serve as the leading reference or text in the field in efforts to close the cancer divide in global oncology care, research, and education.

1.2 Book overview

Harambee in Swahili literally means 'all pull together'. With the growing global burden of cancer and the cancer divide, the emerging consensus is that everyone must pull together via international collaborations in global oncology care, research, and education. Chapter 2 focuses on global oncology education and capacity building with lectures on sustainable initiatives, addressing the dire shortages of health professionals in many parts of the world. It also covers the work of leading oncology professional societies including the American Association for Clinical Oncology (ASCO), the American Society for Therapeutic Radiology (ASTRO), the African Organization for Research and Training in Cancer (AORTIC), and the Federation of African Medical Physicist Organization (FAMPO) amongst others. Chapter 2 concludes with global oncology e-learning platforms and resources.

Following on from education and capacity building, chapter 3 focuses on global oncology research, beginning with the important issue of funding for cancer research, with a lecture from the National Cancer Institute Center for Global Health. This is then followed by ICT for e-research in global oncology. In addition to ICT, this chapter also presents lecture content on smart radiotherapy biomaterials and low-cost technologies for global oncology.

Chapter 4 covers global oncology care, including providing an industry perspective on global oncology from two of the presidents of leading companies looking to participate more actively in closing the cancer divide. Additional perspective is provided from an expert from the International Atomic Energy Agency (IAEA) program in an LMIC. This is followed by lectures on palliative care and the GHC Win–Win Initiative.

In recognition of the old adage that prevention is better than a cure, chapter 5 presents lectures on cancer prevention and advocacy, with highly innovative outreach in collaboration with celebrity athletes, the resource-laden diasporas, and religious institution partners.

In chapter 6, some of the most frequently asked questions in global oncology and radiation oncology are presented with answers from global health leaders. The final chapter reviews the need for and benefit of global oncology collaborations, or Harambee, providing future perspectives on where this growing field will be in the years ahead.

References

[1] Varmus H and Kumar H S 2013 Addressing the growing international challenge of cancer: a multinational perspective *Sci. Transl. Med.* **5** 175

[2] Ngwa W and Ngoma T 2016 *Emerging Models for Global Health in Radiation Oncology* (Bristol: IOP Publishing)

[3] Ngwa W *et al* 2016 Closing the cancer divide through Ubuntu: information and communication technology-powered models for global radiation oncology *Int. J. Rad. Oncol. Biol. Phys.* **94** 440–9

[4] Ngwa W *et al* 2015 Potential for information and communication technologies to catalyze global collaborations in radiation oncology *Int. J. Rad. Oncol. Biol. Phys.* **91** 444–7

[5] Dalal S *et al* 2011 Non-communicable diseases in sub-Saharan Africa: what we know now *Int. J. Epidemiol.* **40** 885–901

Chapter 2

Global oncology education

Vanessa Kerry, Brian D Kavanagh, Nazik Hammad, Bruce Curran, Taofeeq Ige and Wilfred Ngwa

2.1 Seed Global Health

Lecture by Vanessa Kerry (CEO of Seed Global Health); co-edited by Omoruyi Credit Irabor, Juliet Matton, and Wilfred Ngwa.

2.1.1 Introduction

Cancer is on the rise globally, and incidence in the sub-Saharan Africa region is predicted to increase by 85% by 2030 [1]. Overall, case fatality for all cancers is 75% for low income countries in Africa, 72% in its low-middle income countries, and 64% in the upper-middle income countries (collectively the low to middle income countries (LMICs)), significantly higher than the 46% average in high income countries (HICs) [2]. A major contributor to this disparity is the unequal access to healthcare resulting from the shortfall in human resource for health (HRH), fomented by the limited training and leadership capacity of low-resource countries [2]. A need-based analysis in 2013 estimated the world to be short of 17.4 million health workers (including 2.6 million doctors and over 9 million nurses) and forecasts a shortage of 18 million by 2030 [3], affecting both HICs and LMICs [3, 4]. This scarcity has affected health systems across the globe to a varying degree. While the absolute deficits are also significant in South-East Asia due to its population size, the disparity between the global burden of disease and the available healthcare professional workforce is extremely stark in Africa [5]. The continent has 25% of the global burden of disease but only 3% of the world's healthcare workforce. Africa's HRH deficit has led to the emergence of a few not-for-profit companies with the aim to support workforce development within the region. One such initiative is Seed Global Health [6], started in 2011 with a focus to provide nursing and medical training support in resource-constrained countries. Seed Global Health teamed up with the Peace Corps to create the Global Health Service Partnership (GHSP) [7], an initiative that has introduced a novel model for tackling the HRH crises in

doi:10.1088/978-0-7503-1359-9ch2

developing regions of the world. In 2016, Seed Global Health and other stakeholders shared their model of and approach to global health and cancer control at the Global Health Catalyst (GHC) summit at Harvard Medical School. Based on proceedings from the conference, this paper explores the GHSP model for advancing the development of a global health workforce from an oncology perspective, appraising its impact in closing the global cancer care disparity.

2.1.2 The human resource for health crisis in Africa

The 2006 World Health Report indicated 36 of the 57 countries that have a health workforce crisis globally to be in the African region [4]. Although the continent is home to about 11% of the world's population, it has only 3% of global health workers, significantly lower than a region like North America, where the United States and Canada host 37% of the global health workforce for only 14% of the world's population [5]. In 2011, there was an estimated two physicians for every 10 000 people in sub-Saharan Africa, compared to the world average of 15 per 10 000 [8]. The statistics were even gloomier for the nursing profession in Africa, there are 12 nurses per 10 000 people, compared to the world average of 33 per 10 000 [9].

Brain drain is one of the most significant influences for the human resource crisis in sub-Saharan Africa; made up of both 'push' and 'pull' factors, brain drain has been well delineated [10, 11]. Push factors are inherent problems within a country or health system that impede desirable training, employment, and retention incentives for health professionals. These forces include budgetary constraints for health professional education or running the health sector, poor remuneration for health professionals, lack of non-financial incentives such as social recognition, workplace safety, technology, and/or political stability, for example [10, 11]. Pull factors are external to a country or health system, and usually include better standards of living or quality of life, higher salaries, access to advanced technology, and greater political stability in the countries that attract talent from less resourced areas [10, 11]. The costs of this outflow of health workers can be considerable, and also posit an ethical issue [12]. When less resourced nations pay to educate their healthcare workers only to have them leave for developed countries, they are, in effect, subsidizing wealthier nations [12]. A recent analysis estimates the loss of returns from investment for all doctors currently from selected sub-Saharan African countries working in more resourced nations at $2.17 billion, with costs ranging from $2.16 million for Malawi to $1.41 billion for South Africa [12]. Correcting these losses requires a delicate balancing act that protects the right of individual workers to legally migrate, while ensuring that global healthcare needs are met [11]. However, with little incentive for health professionals to migrate from HICs to LMICs, or to remain in LMICs, such a balance might not be easy to achieve.

2.1.3 The Global Health Service Partnership

In a response to this unmet need, Seed Global Health partnered with the US Peace Corps to launch the GHSP. GHSP is an innovative public–private partnership and global health program that sends faculty to medical and nursing schools in under-resourced settings, with the aim to improve the HRH capacity, strengthen global health systems, and ultimately save lives [13]. The GHSP vision and operative model is, in the words of its founders (Kerry, Auld, and Farmer) published prior to its creation in 2012 (although they have expanded the debt repayment beyond educational loans alone), as follows [14]:

> We envision this program as an International Health Service Corps (IHSC), through which health care workers would engage in medical-service and capacity-building partnerships overseas in exchange for health-related graduate school scholarships and forgiveness of student loans. This effort should be targeted to health care providers in the United States and partner countries who are committed to serving the poor.

The GHSP was a landmark in its creation, in part because efforts for such a global health initiative had been underway since former US President John F Kennedy created the Peace Corps by Executive Order in 1961 [15]. In 1979, Senator Javits proposed the International Health Act of 1979, aimed at building an International Health Service program, but it was never passed [16]. The President's Emergency Program for AIDS Relief (PEPFAR), which currently helps fund the GHSP, was itself launched by the US Government in 2003. And in 2005, the Institute of Medicine published a report titled *Healers Abroad: Americans Responding to the Human Resource Crisis in HIV/AIDS*, detailing a Global Health Service Corps that would send health professionals to offer clinical, technical, and managerial support to healthcare workers in developing countries [17]. At that same time, Senator William Frist (R, Tennessee) introduced a bill for a Corps; it failed to progress to legislation.

Few global health advocates, political diplomats, or institutions continued advocacy for a GHSP-model for international health, until the Peace Corps and Seed Global Health (then called Global Health Service Corps) launched GHSP in March 2012. Notable of these advocates are Dr Fitzhugh Mullan (who proposed a model that blended the strengths of the US Peace Corps and the National Health Service Corps [18] and chaired the Institute of Medicine that released reports focusing on the importance of health to international development and diplomacy), Dr Paul Farmer, and Senator Frist.

2.1.4 The GSPH model

The GHSP model works through the recruitment and deployment of doctors and nurses to medical and nursing training institutions in low resource settings, supporting a range of US health professionals to serve as clinical faculty—formally and informally teaching students and house-staff through daily rounds on patients, and separate regularly scheduled didactic sessions and courses [7, 13]. The model aims to enhance existing clinical training systems and structures through the development and implementation of innovative teaching tools, clinical guidelines, treatment protocols, and continuing education programs in partnership with the host country faculty [7, 13]. GHSP volunteers work closely with in-country faculty

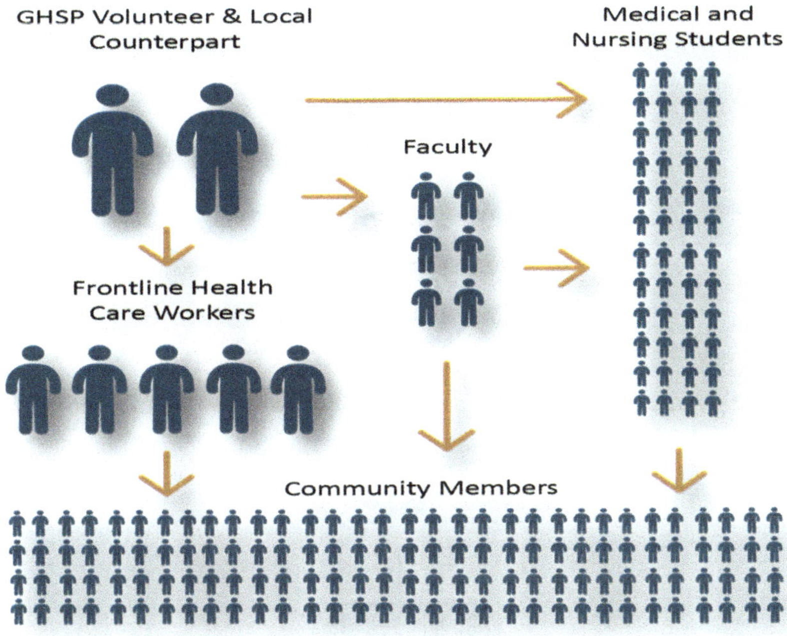

Figure 2.1. The GHSP train the trainer model.

to help ensure they integrate into and foster an efficient and culturally sensitive educational environment (see figure 2.1).

The selection process for GHSP placements is through a consultative process in partnership with the Ministries of Health and of Higher Education, their commitment to strengthening their healthcare systems, a strong in-country PEPFAR presence, and committed local implementing partners [13, 19, 20]. A mapping exercise is undertaken with the US and international partners to reach rapid consensus on priority countries for roll-out of the pilot [19, 20]. GHSP's aim is to create a continuum of health professionals who can teach to the country's disease burden and can serve as educators in the health and education system of their countries (see figure 2.1).

Each cohort of health professionals must include board eligible, or board certified doctors and nurses experienced as educators in core specialties. GHSP volunteers are awarded medical or nursing licenses in the countries where they work to ensure they are fully qualified and approved. To facilitate health professionals to be able to serve, GHSP helps ensure that educational or other debt would not preclude being able to serve. The program, through private philanthropy raised by Seed, provides up to $30 000 of debt repayment for each year served [20]. GHSP is also aiming to create specific partnerships with academic institutions to create a structured sabbatical program and to help recruit mid-career health professionals [20].

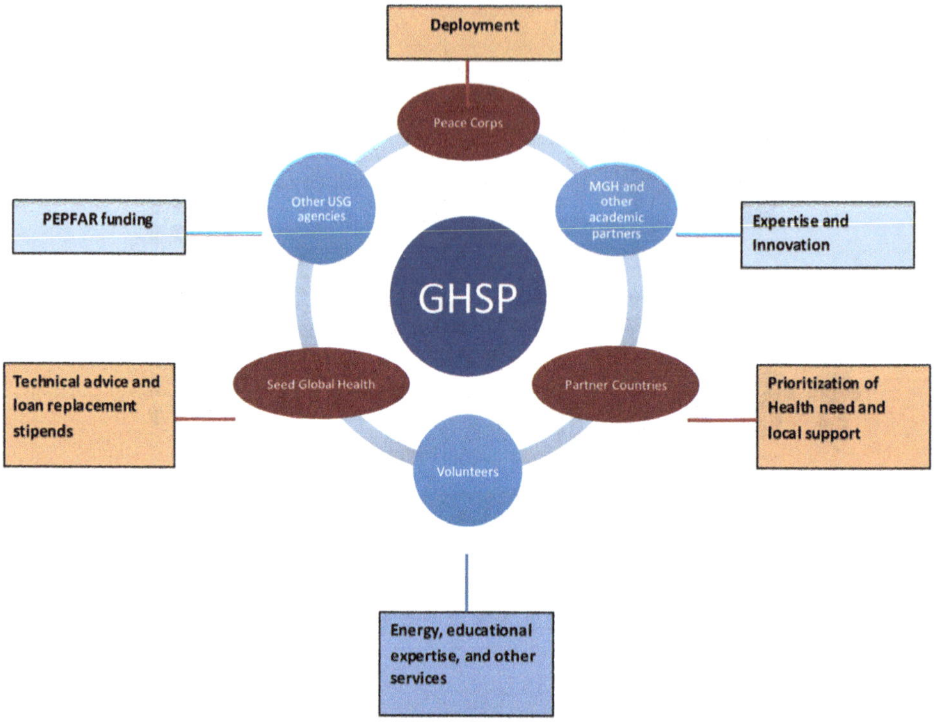

Figure 2.2. The GHSP partnership model [21].

2.1.5 Impact assessment

2.1.5.1 Global health impact

A. **Partnership**

The GHSP has prioritized leveraging partnerships to build and develop the program. GHSP and Seed have received funding from government partners including PEPFAR and the CDC as well as donations from private enterprises, which are raised solely by Seed to support the loan repayment and other critical complementary activities [19, 20]. Peace Corps provides robust experience in sending Americans abroad and helps to handle all administrative needs for the program, building on the economy of scale of its traditional program. Seed Global Health provides technical support and leverages academic, corporate, and other partners to support the program. For example, in collaboration with Massachusetts General Hospital, a Seed flagship academic partner, GSHP awards Fellowships in Global Clinical Education to volunteers at the year's end; the Fellowship recognizes the academic educational experience of the volunteer as well as their contribution in service. Massachusetts General Hospital also supports continuing education credits and provides access to electronic journals and other academic resources.

B. **HRH development**

Seed has assessed GHSP's HRH development using several principle domains: the activities and output of faculty, value added to the learning environment, engaged scholarship, and its ability to empower health workers. These contributions are seen through specific cancer initiatives as well.

1. *GHSP faculty activities and output*

   The program was launched in Tanzania, Malawi, and Uganda in July 2013, at 11 institutions including: the University of Malawi College of Medicine, Mzuzu University, and Kamuzu College of Nursing in Malawi; Gulu University, Lira School of Nursing, and Mbarara University of Science and Technology in Uganda; and the Muhimbili University of Health and Allied Sciences, MVUMI Clinical Officers Training Center, Mirembe School of Nursing, Bugando Medical Center and its affiliate site, Sengerema, in Tanzania. This first cohort consisted of 15 nurses and 16 physicians, selected from a pool of 70 medical and 90 nursing applications [13, 19]. Ten of the 31 volunteers had more than 25 years of clinical experience; seven had between 5 and 15 years of clinical experience, and 14 had less than five years of clinical experience. In the program's first year, GHSP volunteers provided 32 102 h of service, addressing the training needs and human resource gaps of host countries as determined by the countries, and offered 108 courses to 2853 trainees. The second cohort grew to deploy 42 volunteers from a larger pool of applicants, and provided 53 553 h of service, offering 193 courses to 4366 trainees. Halfway through the third year, GHSP had sent a cumulative total of 105 volunteers, and provided a cumulative 104 677 service hours, and 344 courses and training for 9556 trainees (see figures 2.3 and 2.4 and table 2.1) with six months left in the academic year.

2. *Scholarship engagement*

   GHSP has contributed to global cancer care through a partnership between Seed Global Health, the Mbarara University of Science and Technology (MUST) in Uganda, and the Massachusetts General Hospital Cancer Center in the United States, which supports local faculty, residents, and clinical care. MUST is in southwestern Uganda, a region with among the fewest resources and where cancer is a leading cause of death. The university has prioritized creating a cancer center to provide quality diagnosis, treatment, and care for the region. GHSP has responded by sending clinical oncology educators to support scale-up of needed human resources. This contribution also aligns with that of the Massachusetts General Hospital who, also through the GHSP platform, has retained clinical faculty in the oncology specialties, using targeted training opportunities for clinicians and other cancer care-givers across the care continuum [22]. Massachusetts General and Seed have further strengthened human resource development through the

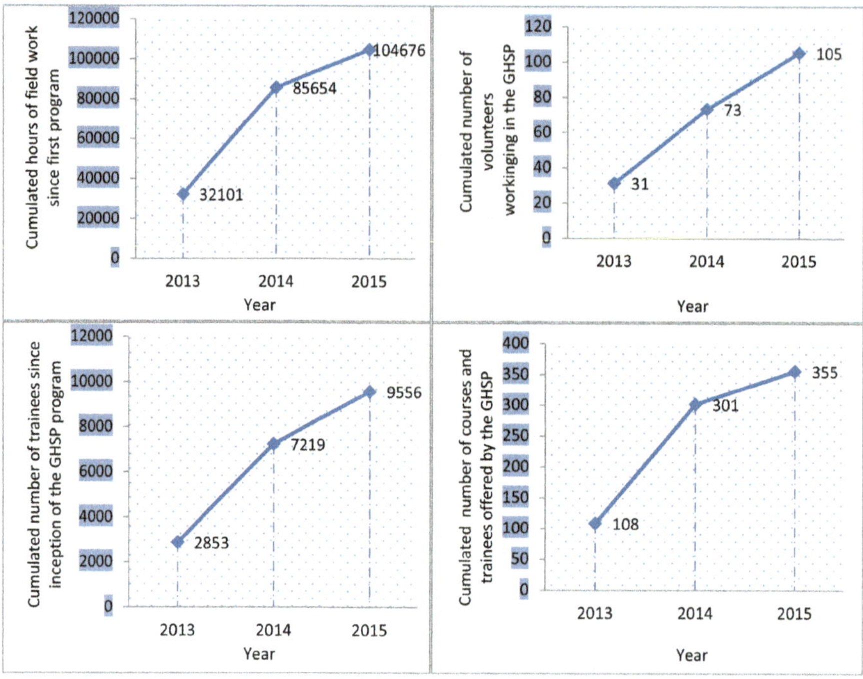

Figure 2.3. Cumulative growth in number of volunteers, service hours, trainees, and courses offered by GHSP.

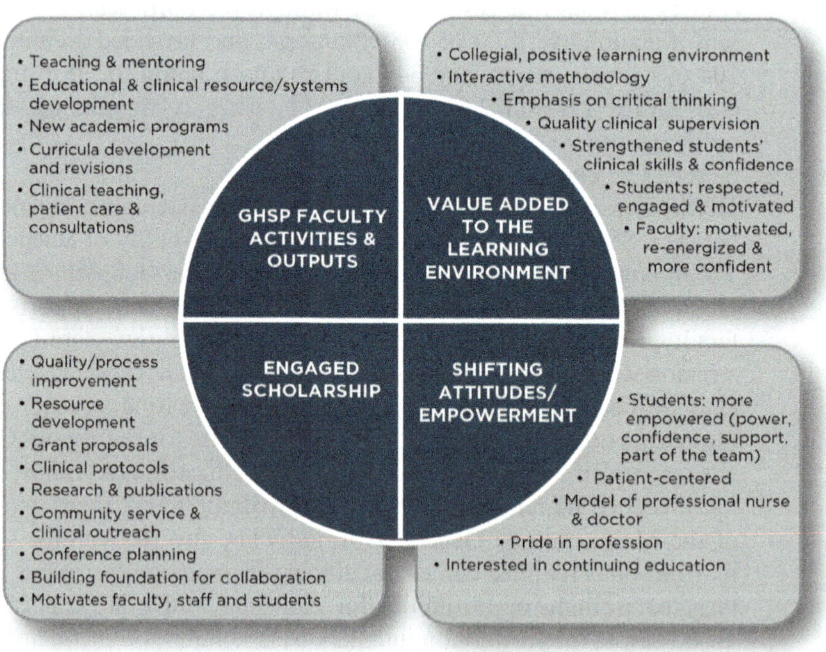

Figure 2.4. Reported GHSP volunteer impact.

Table 2.1. The increasing impact.

	Year 1	Year 2	Year 3	Total
Volunteers	31	42	32	105
Service hours	32 102	53 553	19 022	104 677
Courses and training	108	193	54	355
Trainees	2853	4366	2337*	9556*

*The third year training session was not yet over at the time data was collected.

offering of post-graduate scholarships for physicians and nurses, including in subspecialty clinical fellowships of hematology, surgical oncology, pathology, and global nursing fellowships, and have helped provide clinical physician mentorship (in-person and remote). Seed and Massachusetts General have together invested in pathology training, including scale up of equipment in order to support appropriate diagnosis. Finally, in Tanzania, GHSP has also supported an ongoing collaborative effort with the University of Dodoma and the Tanzanian Ministry of Health to train health providers and professional students on the simple techniques to prevent cervical cancer.

3. *Value added to learning environment and empowerment*
   Qualitative data from in-country student and faculty interviews suggest that the GHSP educator added value to the learning environment through enhanced clinical education, quality clinical supervision, strengthening student clinical skills, critical thinking, and confidence (see figure 2.4). These data suggest that visiting faculty, when vested in a culturally appropriate and locally tailored approach, can contribute to the production of nurses and physicians who are skilled and practice-ready when they graduate (see figure 2.4).
4. *Shifting attitude/empowerment*
   These values contributed to enhance self-reported empowerment, confidence, and pride in the profession as health providers see themselves as competent and capable of delivery health solutions [13, 19]. These data suggest that visiting faculty in a culturally appropriate and locally tailored manner to serve in partnership with country department can contribute to the production of nurses and physicians who are skilled and practice-ready when they graduate (see figure 2.4).

C. **Infrastructural development**
GHSP has provided support for infrastructure improvement, recognizing that adequate tools are needed for teaching and for health professionals to practice in what they train. Specific to cancer care, GHSP has made

contributions to cancer care in partnership with Massachusetts General, including supporting core equipment for pathology training. Seed also nurtured a relationship with the American Society for Clinical Pathology (ASCP) and Butaro University in Rwanda to see modest, targeted infrastructural upgrades for cancer diagnosis and management that include microscopes and telepathology in Rwanda. The ASCP initiative mainly aims to improve the accuracy and clinical relevance of cancer diagnosis in African settings. GHSP, through scholarships for MMed, direct mentorships, and training, has concurrently supported human resource capability to ensure laboratory upgrades are well utilized. These efforts complement again those of Massachusetts General, which has helped with the construction of pediatric and adult in-patient wards, infusion chairs, and biosecurity fume hoods for chemotherapy preparation.

2.1.5.2 Impact in the US

Global health initiatives such as GHSP could immensely benefit the US economy and health system. According to the Pew Research Center, The US population is projected to rise to 438 million in 2050, from 296 million in 2005, and 82% of the increase will be due to immigrants arriving from 2005 to 2050 and their US-born descendants [23]. Of the projected 117 million people added to the population during this period due to the effect of new immigration, 67 million will be the immigrants themselves and 50 million will be their US-born children or grandchildren [23]. There is thus an increasing need for US physicians and educators to acquire the knowledge, attitudes, and skills needed to help care for the diversity of these individuals [24–26]. In recognition of the diverse, global population in the country, US medical and nursing education is already promoting inclusivism in the classroom through multicultural teaching and providing culturally competent care to their patients [24–26]. GHSP provides a meaningful cross-cultural experience which develops clinical skills, exposes participants to a broad spectrum of diseases, and encourages them to work in under-served specialties or under-served areas in the US [24–26].

2.1.6 Future perspective

The GHSP program plans to continue its expansion. Plans are underway (at the time of presentation) to launch GHSP into five countries in total, including Liberia and Swaziland, and plans to double the number of volunteers in each country are already underway. GHSP is a necessary model to help counter the growing need for health professionals globally.

2.2 The American Society for Radiation Oncology (ASTRO)

Lecture by Brian D Kavanagh (President of ASTRO); lecture notes co-edited by Neharika Sinha and W Ngwa.

2.2.1 Introduction

Radiotherapy is a complex but cost-effective means of treating cancer and relieving symptoms. Developing countries possess only one third of the world's radiotherapy equipment, in spite of the fact that they constitute 85% of the world's population. A survey of 20 LMICs found one radiotherapy unit to every 5 million people and, sometimes, one unit for every 20 million people. Currently, many countries do not have a single radiotherapy machine, with seven out of ten cancer deaths globally occurring in developing countries. The American Society of Radiation Oncology (ASTRO) aims to expand the role of radiation oncologists in achieving more equitable healthcare for all global citizens through collaborative humanitarian outreach, education, and research [27, 28]. A tremendous effort to bridge the radiotherapy gap is being made.

However, good intentions, even with lots of money, do not guarantee better healthcare in a developing country. The Cornwall Regional Hospital was the first multidisciplinary hospital constructed in Jamaica since the building of the University Hospital 21 years before. At the time it was considered one of the most elaborate and sophisticated institutions of its kind in the world. It was the largest single investment made by the Jamaican government. It followed the American model of a high-cost, hospital-centered healthcare delivery system that led to the commitment of the largest capital investment ever in the health sector. Investment in this institution by the World Bank created very serious demands on the Jamaican health budget, as there were many design faults. The design placed a boiler under the casualty department to provide heating during the winter. Jamaica does not have a winter season and the heat of the Jamaican summer became so unbearable that the department had to be abandoned during the summer. This example illustrates the need for developing optimal models for each country. The current consensus is that US/European models are not always optimal.

In view of all of these, ASTRO is making efforts in several international global healthcare programs. This paper highlights some of ASTRO's initiatives, with a plan to determine the unique optimal model for each region or country.

2.2.2 ASTRO international activities for global health

2.2.2.1 The International Education Committee

Pre-2011, ASTRO international activities included: a breakfast for international attendees at the annual meeting; random, occasional sponsorship of speakers at international meetings; and activities by members who independently were starting good programs and developing relationships. Then the International Education Committee (IEC), aka the International Education Subcommittee Task Force, was established by ASTRO in 2010. This led to the development of a strategic plan for radiation oncology worldwide. An example from the 2012 report on South-East Asia is given in table 2.2.

It became obvious that while many centers in these LMICs have modern equipment, including IMRT, IGRT, SRS, and SBRT, the training for the use of

Table 2.2. Status of radiation oncology in five South-East Asian countries.

	Indonesia	Malaysia	Philippines	Singapore	Thailand
Radiation oncologists	41	52	55	30	95
Physicists	43	48	36	20	83
Technicians	133	198	100	94	190
RT Centers	20	22	31	5	28
LINACs/Co60	15/16	33/2	17/10	16/0	39/22

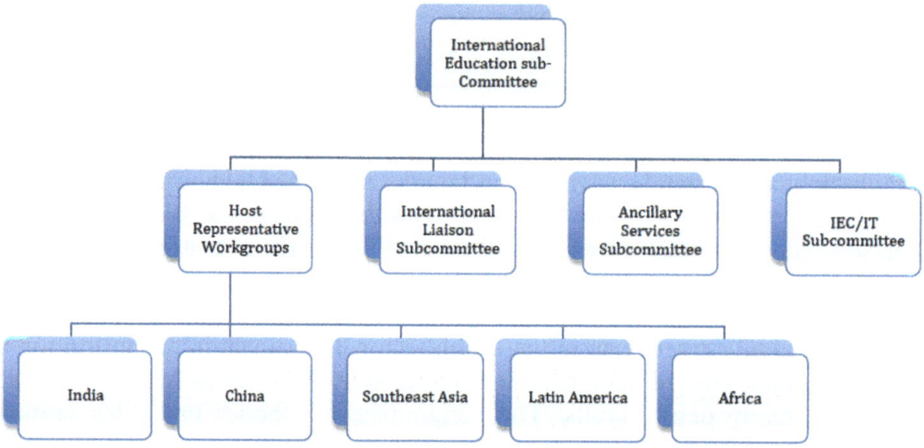

Figure 2.5. Illustration of the structure emerging from the recommendations.

these advanced technologies is very limited. On the other hand, many countries have equipment which is outdated and insufficient.

The 2012 ASTRO Task Force recommendations included the creation of five workgroups, for India, China, Southeast Asia, Latin America, and Africa. Each workgroup was charged with creating a specific plan for assessing needs, establishing goals, deploying ASTRO resources, and developing region-specific metrics to assess progress. Another recommendation was the creation of an IEC International Liaison Subcommittee to ensure that ASTRO members are also in ESTRO, IAEA, NCI/NIH, ASCO, JASTRO, RANZCR, TASTRO, and SASCRO, with the goal of collaborating with other societies to build bridges between international societies. Another recommendation was the creation of an Ancillary Services Subcommittee, constituting ASTRO members who are also members of the AAPM, AAMD, ASRT, and ARON, in order to coordinate and harmonize the efforts of the IEC with these specialties. An IEC/IT workgroup was also created to take care of technical matters. See figure 2.5 for an illustration of the structure.

2.2.2.2 The ASTRO/ARRO Global Health Scholars (GHS) program

The Global Health Scholars (GHS) program, formally launched in 2011, was designed to allow senior residents interested in global health an opportunity to work on a resident-designed clinical, outreach/educational, or research project in a developing nation. This program also intends to foster a global perspective of oncology and encourage ongoing outreach, research and progress in developing countries.

2.2.2.3 The International Education Committee 2.0

In 2013, ASTRO International Education Subcommittee presented a Progress Report and was reorganized. A Special Interest workgroup was newly added in the year 2013. Meanwhile, the five regional Work Groups were charged to make an assessment of the educational needs with the following top three priorities:

- Technology assessment: treatment delivery and planning QA.
- Ancillary services: therapists, physicists, dosimetrists, nurses, support staff.
- IT infrastructure across each region and methods of information exchange.

In the proposed strategy there were also three top priorities: to develop overall strategies to improve education in the region, identify three ways ASTRO can improve education (in order of priority), and develop metrics to track educational success.

The table below shows an example of the early observations and assessment of educational needs for Africa by the Africa workgroup. The top priorities identified for the Africa region are:

a. Establishing direct contact/relationships with centers in countries other than those with well-established programs.
b. The need for collaboration with AAPM to enhance medical physics training.
c. The need for ASTRO resources for Ministries of Health in nations with limited or no radiation therapy.

Table 2.3. Educational needs for radiation oncologists in Africa [28]. Based on a report by Brian D Kavanagh at the 2016 Global Health Catalyst Summit.

Technology assessments	Ancillary services	IT infrastructure
Cobalt remains predominant	Staffing often extremely 'skeletal'	Highly variable
Need to translate advances in RT planning into Cobalt platform	Training non-uniform, need for: – appropriate training for brachytherapy	Resides with Hospitals and Ministries of Health
Need for an AAPM Africa subcommittee	– appropriate training for advanced techniques	Access to Web based accredited training program lectures
Brachytherapy (BT) needs assessment	No formal training, certification and CME for therapists	Institutional relationships with US centers (host-relationships)
Emerging: QA for image guidance	Need for training in Physics, calibration technology and maintenance	

2.2.3 Common perceived need in all regions: education hubs

A common need identified in all regions is that of regional centers which can serve as hubs across their region to disseminate educational content. As an example, Mekelle University is a higher education and training public institution located in the city of Mekelle, Ethiopia, which is expected to have site coordinators and develop into a regional center. Another example is Hunan University, in Changsha, China, ranked number seven in a national survey for all cancer hospitals. As highlighted in the book *Emerging Models for Global Health in Radiation Oncology* [29], one could build collaborations or partnerships with such regional education hubs. The partnership between Botswana and the University of Pennsylvania, and the effort by the University of Wisconsin–Madison and the people of Uganda in East Africa, are just a couple of reference examples.

In establishing educational hubs, the educational methods need to be well organized (see figure 2.6). There could be traditional lectures, through regional or national meetings and institutional events. There could be seminars and hands-on workshops (e.g. on e-contouring, brachytherapy) round table discussions, and colloquia. Webinars on e-contouring, or remote tumor boards and round table discussion could also be valuable. Institutional didactic courses and archived educational or scientific content could be provided as virtual content, i.e. online. Educational manuals covering curriculum development and training standards would also be a great resource. Some examples of existing educational manuals include: *Recommendations for a Global Curriculum in Medical Oncology* by the European Society for Medical Oncology [30] and the *International Atomic Energy Agency Syllabus for the Education and Training of Radiation Oncologists*, endorsed by ASTRO [31] and the European Society for Therapeutic Radiology and Oncology (ESTRO) [31].

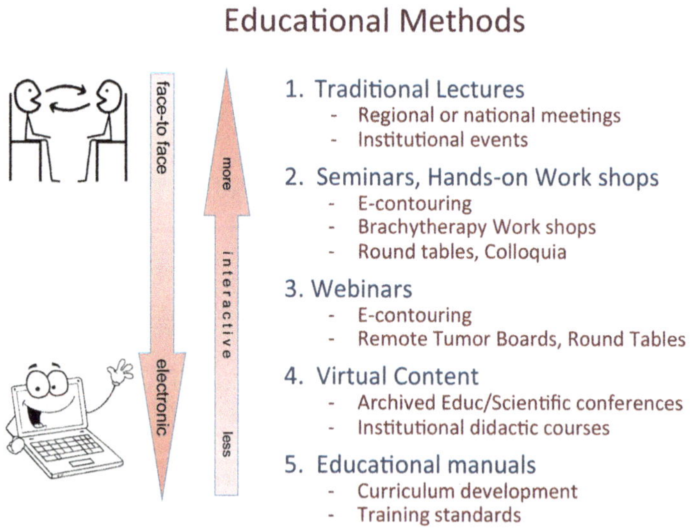

Figure 2.6. Educational methods for global oncology.

Identifying the metrics of success is important and this could be different for every situation. Such metrics could include clinical outcomes, which are monitored through changes in morbidity and mortality. The changes or successes of a process, or organizational outcomes, may also be another metric to be observed through: changes in access to care, such as the number of patients with cancer receiving radiation therapy; changes in type of care, such as the number of patients receiving 3D conformal therapy; and changes in quality of care, such as improvements in the clinical efficiency.

It is essential to also keep in mind that international education is a two-way street, which means developed countries also benefit.

2.2.4 2015 highlights

The highlights of the IES in 2015 included two 90 min educational sessions during the ASTRO annual meeting about how US methods could be adapted in LMICs. The summary courses are also available in Mandarin and Spanish. There was also a presentation by the Union for International Cancer Control (UICC) Collaboration on the Global Task Force on Radiotherapy for Cancer Control (GTFRCC). There is the need for the survey to be incorporated into the survey of Africa to be discussed, as well as a database of international centers for resident elective rotations. In the eContouring initiative, ambassadors travelled to train international practitioners in Armenia, Mexico, Southeast Asia, and Argentina. Finally the iTreatSafely website was launched with a mission to improve quality and safety in radiation therapy by offering high-quality learning videos that deliver practical clinical and QA skills.

There were several other 2015 IES workgroup activities. In an effort to spread the most important science related to radiation oncology throughout the world, ASTRO has created a program that allows organizations to license the Best of ASTRO content and hold an officially licensed live meeting in their own country. This was done in Latin America (in Mexico) and the annual meeting courses were presented in Spanish. A live meeting was also held in India and the resultant survey was published [33]. There was a Mandarin refresher course at the annual meeting and various web-based educational activities by the Chinese workgroup. The Southeast Asia group held a Plans for Best of ASTRO session at a Federation of Asian Organizations in Radiation Oncology (FARO) meeting. There were also other activities in Botswana and Turkey.

Looking forward, there is significant ongoing effort to develop the Chartrounds international society for improving cancer care. With chartrounds.com, patient management and treatment plans are analyzed with trusted cancer experts in real time. Chartrounds brings together academic disease site specialists from leading cancer treatment institutions and connects them with the Chartrounds network of over 1500 physicians and medical physicists. It currently covers 34 countries with 85 global members.

2.2.5 Conclusions

According to WHO, cancer is currently one of the leading causes of morbidity and mortality worldwide. Annual incidence of cancer is expected to rise by 70% in developing countries over the next two decades. These numbers are alarming and pose a great threat to the well-being of those living in developing countries. Ongoing efforts by ASTRO are important to help address this threat, including via The ARRO Global Health Initiative, the International Education Committee, collaborations with other societies, and building bridges between international societies.

'All international education efforts and cultural exchange are based on personal relationships.' (Brian Kavanagh, MD (President of ASTRO), April 29, 2017, Boston, MA).

2.3 The African Organization for Research and Training in Cancer (AORTIC)

Lecture by Nazik Hammad (Vice President of AORTIC North America); lecture notes co-edited by Wilfred Ngwa.

2.3.1 Introduction

The African Organization for Research and Training in Cancer (AORTIC) was formed in 1983 by expatriate African cancer care workers, scientists, and their friends, and is dedicated to the promotion of cancer control in Africa. AORTIC's key objectives are to further the research relating to cancers prevalent in Africa, support the management of training programs in oncology for healthcare workers, deal with the challenges of creating cancer control and prevention programs, and raise public awareness of cancer in Africa. Through its Education and Training Committee, AORTIC aims to provide and facilitate high quality cancer education and training for African cancer clinicians, researchers, advocates, survivors, policy makers, and students.

The importance of education and training for cancer health professionals from Africa cannot be over-emphasized with medical oncology training having a vital impact on patient care (figure 2.7). Currently teachers or faculty are a scare resource. Available faculty have significant demands related to service, leadership, and teaching, contrasted with poor compensation and poor resources for faculty development—'train the trainer'. Some of this results in brain drain, which further exacerbates the situation.

To address this situation, AORTIC Education and Training Committee goals include to:

- Establish the AORTIC Virtual Education & Training Program.
- Implement Centers of Excellence in Cancer Education & Training that address all areas of the cancer control continuum Goal of Interest.
- Improve human capacity building and workforce diversity through the education and training of multidisciplinary specialists.
- Develop curriculum for specialty training, certificate courses, and postgraduate training programs.
- Partner with international and continental organizations to organize regional meetings.

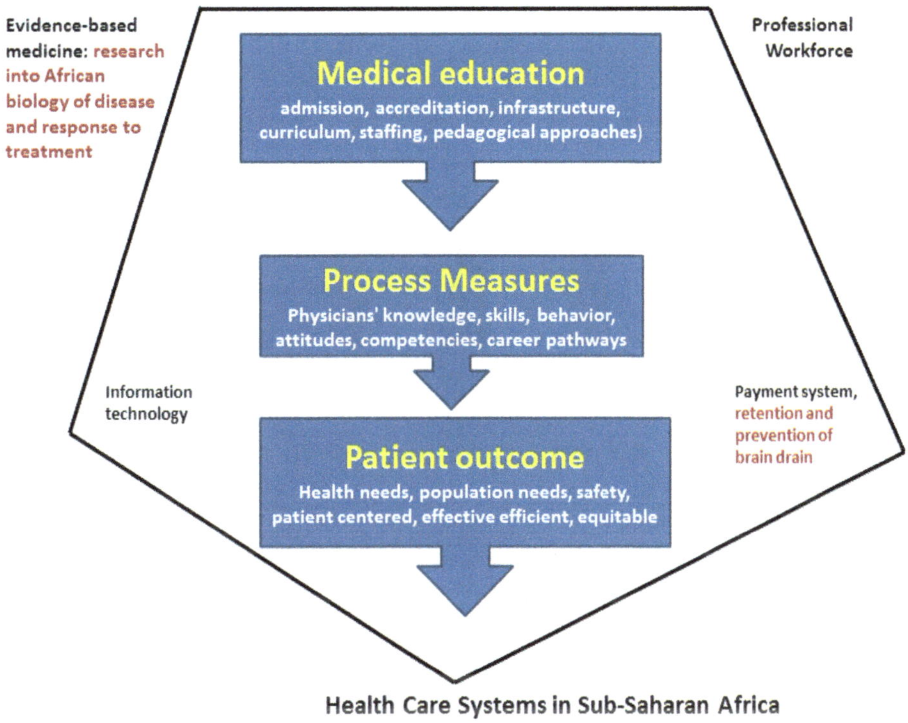

Figure 2.7. Model of the effect of the medical education continuum upon patient outcomes [34].

2.3.2 Virtual education and training program

AORTIC has officially launched its virtual education and training platform as part of AORTIC's leading efforts dedicated to building capacity for cancer control in Africa. The online education and training platform was developed by the AORTIC Education and Training Committee in consonance with AORTIC's dedication to the promotion of cancer control and palliation in Africa for over 25 years. The platform is designed to facilitate and support training initiatives in oncology for healthcare workers, helping build human capacity for cancer control in Africa for the twenty-first century and beyond. The online educational platform is free for any AORTIC member and aims to expand cancer education and training opportunities to anyone with an internet connection and a smartphone or computer. The courses with certificates offered on the platform highly complement other cancer education and training efforts by AORTIC and partners. AORTIC offers certificate courses via the platform but also provides links to partner platforms with complementary online education and training content.

The launch of this platform follows on the heels of a burgeoning information and communications technology sector in Africa. In a recent survey of hundreds of healthcare professionals in Africa (figure 2.8) it was found that over 86% have a

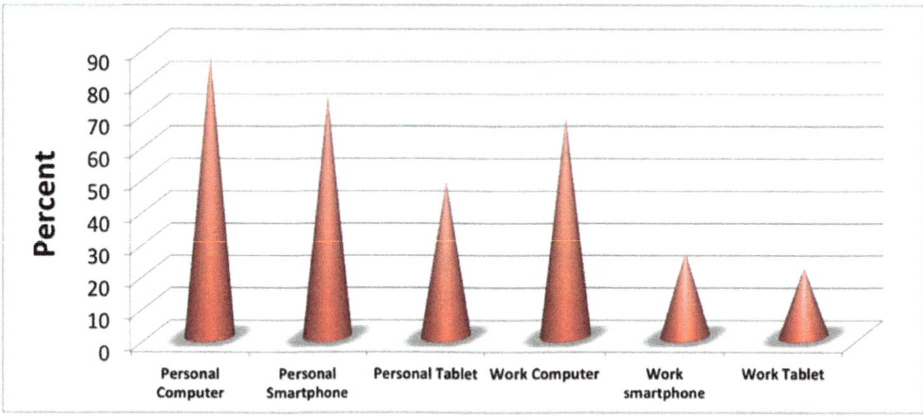

Figure 2.8. Access to information technology tools needed for online learning among healthcare professionals in Africa.

personal computer and 75% a personal smartphone. This means that many can now take courses online.

In 2017, a number of courses have been planned for delivery using the AORTIC online learning platform. These courses include: the basics of mixed methods research certificate program, global radiation oncology, psycho-oncology, clinical trials, molecular pathology, basic and translational research, medical oncology, and advocacy. AORTIC is well positioned to lead the education of cancer healthcare professionals in an increasingly interdependent continent and an interdependent world. Leading activities include: a continent-wide strategic plan for education of oncology healthcare professionals; accreditation of educational content; addressing equity and health needs; coordination and collaboration with the American Society for Clinical Oncology and the European Society for Clinical Oncology, and other organizations; and support of educational scholarships and research to assess existing training programs and educational initiatives, as well as new and emerging ones. AORTIC welcomes new members to help chart the future in cancer research and education in Africa in the years ahead.

2.4 The American Association for Physicists in Medicine (AAPM): international outreach programs

Lecture by Bruce Curran (President, American Association of Physicists in Medicine)

2.4.1 Introduction

The American Association of Physicists in Medicine (AAPM) was founded in 1958. It is a scientific and professional organization, and currently has 8839 members in 97 countries. The mission of the AAPM is to advance the science, education, and professional practice of medical physics, a broad-based scientific and professional discipline that encompasses physical principles with applications in biology and medicine. The clinical practice is dedicated to ensuring accuracy, safety, and quality in the use of radiation in medical procedures such as medical imaging and radiation therapy.

The AAPM provides a variety of programs, membership opportunities, and resources for medical physicists, students, and related medical and scientific professionals anywhere in the world. The goals of the AAPM are to promote the highest quality medical physics services for patients, and encourage research and development to advance the discipline. AAPM disseminates scientific and technical information in the discipline, fosters the education and professional development of medical physicists, supports the medical physics education of physicians and other medical professionals, promotes standards for the practice of medical physics, and governs and manages the Association in an effective, efficient, and fiscally responsible manner. Medical physicists are concerned with clinical service and consultation, research and development, and teaching.

2.4.2 AAPM international efforts

The AAPM members are involved in other organizations, such as the International Organization for Medical Physics (IOMP), The Canadian Organization of Medical Physicists (COMP), the European Society for Radiation Oncology (ESTRO), European Federation of Organizations for Medical Physics (EFOMP), Medical Physics for World Benefit (MPWB), International Atomic Energy Agency (IAEA), and other national and regional societies. The AAPM programs are a collaborative effort. As an international effort the AAPM is consolidated into two major committees, the International Educational Activities Committee (IEAC) and the International Affairs Committee (IAC).

The IEAC ensures that AAPM provides medical physics educational programs and educational resources to medical physicists working outside the USA and Canada, and coordinates between these international educational activities of the AAPM and those of related organizations.

The committee has the following functions:

- Assess, periodically, the need for international educational activities and the associated activities of the AAPM.
- Develop and maintain policies for allocation of the AAPM's international educational resources.
- Develop and maintain policies for the conduct of AAPM's international education activities.
- Plan, develop, and direct, as appropriate, the international educational programs and activities of the AAPM, including the International Scientific Exchange Program (ISEP).
- Coordinate the educational activities of the AAPM with those of related organizations.
- Endorse and co-sponsor non-AAPM international education activities.
- Recommend to the AAPM Board sponsorship of non-AAPM international education activities.

- Provide advice to international organizations about educational needs in medical physics.
- Recommend to the AAPM Board advice intended for international agencies and foreign governments about the educational needs in medical physics.
- Develop budgets for the international educational activities of the AAPM.

Meanwhile the mission of the AAPM IAC is to advise the AAPM Board of Directors through the Administrative Council on matters related to activities of an international nature conducted either by individuals or committees on behalf of the Association. The aim of the IAC is to promote the application of physics to medicine and biology internationally. The committee disseminates scientific, technical, professional, and historical information concerning medical physics internationally. It serves as a clearinghouse for activities of an international nature of members, councils, and committees in order to provide coordination, and makes recommendations to the President-Elect and/or the President for appointments of delegates and alternate delegates to international organizations, such as the International Organization for Medical Physics (IOMP). The committee is also responsible for preparing reports on the international activities of the Association for the Board of Directors through the Administrative Council. Figure 2.9 shows the structure of the IAC.

2.4.3 The International Portal

The International Portal section on the AAPM website www.aapm.org gives guidance on the available resources. This website is open to all, but some specific programs and resources are restricted to AAPM members. Many of the Educational Resources are also available to medical physicists in developing countries. Access requires registration as a Developing Country Educational Associate (DCEA) and obtaining a Developing Country Educational Associate identity.

The website is updated with the list of developing countries recognized by the AAPM. The AAPM/IOMP Library Program serves as a resource for medical physics and related communities in developing countries. The AAPM has a web-based Virtual Library, which contains many of the Continuing Education Courses presented at the AAPM annual meetings. The AAPM members have access to the proceedings of the AAPM Summer Schools. The reports of the many AAPM Groups are available to all. The Equipment Donation Sub-Committee serves the joint partnership between AAPM and IOMP, and works to ensure that available, working-order equipment is put to good use at clinics or educational institutions in LMICs.

AAPM supports its mission by disseminating scientific and technical information in the discipline of medical physics. The AAPM has long advocated a consistent level of medical physics practice, and has published many guidelines and position statements toward that goal, such as: Science Council Task Group reports related to calibration and quality assurance; Education Council and Professional Council Task Group reports related to education, training and peer review; and Board-approved

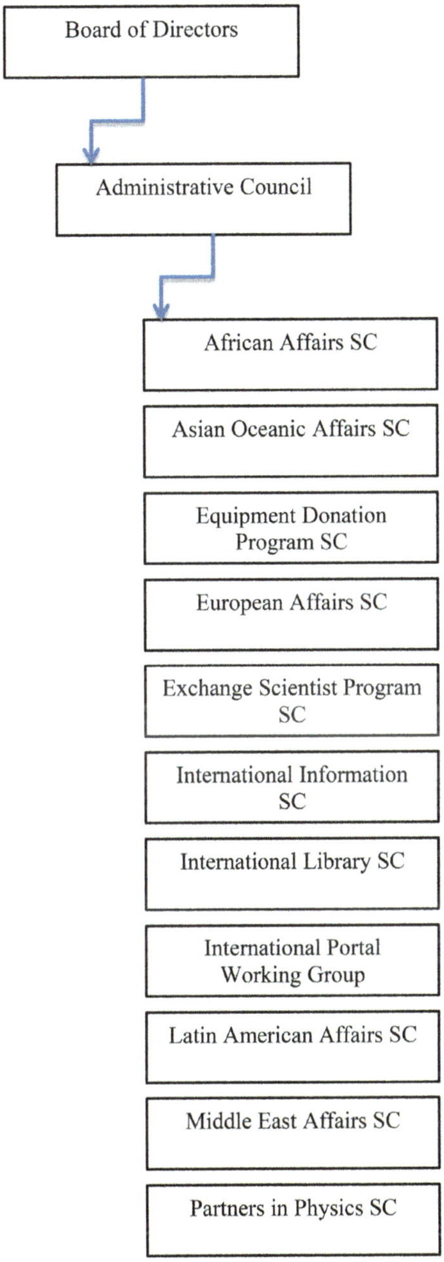

Figure 2.9. Structure of IAC.

position statements related to the scope of practice, physicist qualifications, and other aspects of medical physics practice.

AAPM supports its mission by disseminating scientific and technical information in the discipline of medical physics. Among a number of publications by AAPM, the most highly rated journals are *Medical Physics* and the *Journal of Applied Clinical Medical Physics*.

The AAPM/IOMP Library Program serves as a resource for medical physics and related communities in developing countries. The library program accepts book and e-journal donations and forwards them to established libraries on a per-request basis.

As of November 2014, current participation in the program involves 36 libraries located in 27 countries on five continents. The International Library Subcommittee (ILSC), a subset of the IAC, administers the AAPM portion of the library program.

Medical physicists from developing countries can register to become a DCEA, which provides free and open access to certain educational resources, including proceedings of the AAPM Summer Schools, Continuing Education Programs from the annual meetings, and Selected AAPM Task Group reports.

The Exchange Scientist Program provides an opportunity for members of the AAPM to visit other countries to promote the exchange of scientific information and to facilitate the advancement of the field of medical physics at the international level. The program primarily serves as an information exchange forum by maintaining a list of approved Exchange Scientists (ES) as well as a list, if any, of host institutions interested in requesting an ES for any project. Any subsequent arrangement or contract is entirely between the ES and the host institution, and the ES program in general has no funding or further involvement with the visit, other than publishing the report from the ES on completion of the visit. A further intent of the program is to provide the ES with the status and motivation to pay short visits to other institutions when travelling for business or personal purposes.

The Partners in Physics Program (PIP) provides opportunities for physicists in developing countries to have their application fee and dues waived. For information about the PIP contact the AAPM IAC using the message form for the IAC at the bottom of the AAPM website page.

AAPM provides, sponsors, or co-sponsors a variety of educational and training programs in cooperation with medical physics organizations throughout the world. Each year the ISEP provides continuing education courses on both therapeutic and diagnostic imaging physics in selected developing countries. IEAC administers the international education programs.

2.5 The Federation of African Medical Physics Organizations (FAMPO)

Lecture presented by Taofeeq Ige, (Secretary General of FAMPO)

2.5.1 Introduction

Africa is the world's second largest and second most populous continent. With one billion inhabitants, it accounts for about 15% of the world's human population. It has 54 fully recognized sovereign states, with 49 being United Nations members. Thirty-eight countries are International Atomic Energy Agency (IAEA) member states. Algeria is the largest African country by area and Nigeria is the largest by population. The Federation of African Medical Physics Organizations (FAMPO) was created to be a leading medical physics organization in Africa with the following goals:

- To promote improved quality service to patients and the community in the region.
- To promote co-operation and communication between medical physics organizations in the region and, where such organizations do not exist, between individual medical physicists.
- To promote the profession and practice of medical physics and related activities.
- To promote the advancement in status and standard of practice of the medical physics profession.
- To promote and improve the training of medical physicists.
- To promote research and development in the field of medical physics.
- To promote appropriate use of technology to the benefit of rural populations.
- To organize and/or sponsor international conferences, and regional and other meetings.
- To collaborate or affiliate with other scientific organizations.
- The activities of the Federation are not aimed at profit.

The role of FAMPO in the promotion of education and training programs in Africa include:

- Establishment of an inventory of institutes delivering academic programs.
- Establishment of an inventory of institutes delivering clinical training programs.
- Drafting accreditation criteria for academic and clinical training programs.
- Drafting certification criteria for the medical physics profession.
- Organizing activities to support CPD of the medical physics profession.
- Launching a regional journal on medical physics.

2.5.2 African radiology

Most countries have only basic radiology equipment, 20 countries have access to nuclear medicine. In general fewer medical physicists are dedicated to imaging than to radiotherapy. High-end imaging (e.g. mammography, MRI, PET/CT) is available in the public sector in ten countries. Tele-radiology is limited by telecommunications infrastructure. Twenty-five countries have radiotherapy facilities and 12 out of this 25 have one center. Fewer than ten countries have adequate facilities to service their populations, i.e. a manageable waiting list. A detailed analysis of the status of radiotherapy in Africa could be summarized as follows.

Twenty-eight countries do not have radiotherapy services, 14 have three or fewer machines, and only seven have more than ten machines. Cobalt machines represent ~30% of the equipment. There is an average of 3.8 million people per machine, which varies a lot between different income groups. Between 22% and 28% of the needs are covered depending on the benchmark used. Countries without radiotherapy are slowly setting up their first departments. Sustainability is a problem and expansion is mainly happening in countries with a larger number of machines. Only three countries (Egypt, Morocco, Republic of South Africa) account for more than 50% of qualified medical physicists in the region. Seventy-five per cent of medical physicists are government employees with at least 30% of medical physicists being female.

2.5.3 African medical physicists

Medical physics baseline data in Africa is now available and can gradually be improved upon. The present work contributes in developing a reliable database which will be the formal reference for competent agencies in an attempt to create harmony in the use of resources that will be invested in the continent. The database will help in planning for future programs and launching projects that could be of benefit to all the medical physicists in the region and beyond (see tables 2.4 and 2.5).

Table 2.4. African medical physicist data summary table (RT = radiotherapy, MP = medical physicist, T = temporary, F = full time, population in millions).

COUNTRIES	POPULATION	RT CENTRES	MP(T)	MP(F)
ALGERIA	39	7	39	19
ANGOLA	24	2	4	
BOTSWANA	2	2	4	
BURKINA FASO	17	–	2	–
BURUNDI	9	–	–	–
CAMEROON	19	2	3	1
CHAD	13	–	–	–
COTE D'IVOIRE	24	–	1	–
DEM. REP. CONGO	69			
EGYPT	88	56	150	80
ERITREA	5	–	–	–
ETHIOPIA	88	1	5	0
GABON	2	1	3	0
GHANA	27	3	30	3
KENYA	43	2	8	0
LIBYA	6			
MADAGASCAR	22	1	2	2
MALAWI	16	–	–	–
MALI	17	1	–	–
MAURITANIA	3.5	1	3	0
MAURITIUS	1.2	1	5	1
MOROCCO	34	15	56	22
NAMIBIA	2	1	3	1

Table 2.5. Number of medical physicists per country in Africa.

Country	# of MPs
Algeria	70
Angola	4
Botswana	4
Burkina Faso	2
Burundi	–
Cameroon	3
Chad	–
Cote D'Ivoire	–
Dem. Rep. of the Congo	1
Egypt	183
Ethiopia	3
Gabon	4
Ghana	30
Kenya	8
Libya	27
Madagascar	2
Mali	1[a]
Mauritania	6
Mauritius	4
Morocco	56
Namibia	3
Niger	2
Nigeria	70
Senegal	2
South Africa	130
Sudan	28
Tanzania	6
Tunisia	17
Uganda	5
Zambia	4
Zimbabwe	8

[a]Chinese citizen in Mali (1 MP and 1 therapeutic radiographers).

2.5.4 Implementation constraints

Constraints that need to be taken seriously into account include the fact that the legislation and regulatory framework for radiation protection are often lacking or poor. Also, many countries do not have adequate radiation safety infrastructure in place, and lack a radiation safety culture. There is also a shortage in the quantity and the quality of professionals using radiation in medicine. Currently, there are also no referral guidelines for medical imaging. Obsolete or second-hand equipment without traceable quality control is also an issue. Radiation safety modules in education and training syllabi need to be constantly updated, because even those using radiation lack awareness of the risks of using radiation in medicine. The FAMPO is committed to advancing the implementation of the 10 actions of Bonn Call for Action. These ten actions include:

- Enhancing implementation of justification of procedures.
- Enhancing implementation of optimization of protection and safety.
- Strengthening manufacturers' contribution to radiation safety.
- Strengthening radiation protection education and training of health professionals.
- Shaping and promoting a strategic research agenda for radiation protection in medicine.
- Improving data collection on radiation exposures of patients and workers.
- Improving primary prevention of incidents and adverse events.
- Strengthening radiation safety culture in healthcare.
- Fostering an improved radiation benefit-risk-dialogue.
- Strengthening the implementation of safety requirements (BSS) globally.

Acknowledgements

The author is grateful to the following people and organizations: the IAEA for the improvement of radiotherapy, digital radiography, nuclear medicine, and medical physics in Africa; Professors F Nuesslin, S Tabakov, M Rehani, D van der Merwe, and Dr A Meghzifene; Professor Wilfred Ngwa and the GHCCS team; his FAMPO ExCom—Ahmed, Rebecca, and Odette; and Mr Ernest Nwabueze (Offenburg, GER).

2.6 Other global oncology education initiatives

by Wilfred Ngwa

With membership in over 100 countries, the American Association for Clinical Oncology (ASCO) is the world's largest and arguably most influential oncology organization committed to advancing the frontiers of cancer research, providing excellent educational opportunities, and defining standards of practice for oncology care, while also influencing public policy. ASCO implements international programs focused on supporting oncologic skills training, developing clinical capacity at strategic LMIC hospitals, and supporting the next generation of oncology leaders in LMICs.

2.6.1 Supporting oncologic skills training

ASCO works with institutions across the world to train doctors, nurses, and other clinicians on topics deemed by its partners to be critical to improving cancer outcomes in their countries. Courses offered include cancer control in primary care courses, multidisciplinary cancer management courses, international palliative care courses, and international clinical trials workshops (ICTW). ASCO has launched an ASCO University portal with the mission to provide a comprehensive eLearning Center that supports lifelong learning. As part of ASCO University, there is a learning resource called ASCO-SEP that can be used for self-study. A printed text is accompanied by an eBook version which contains all of the learning content. Once the book is purchased, one may complete the self-assessment and evaluation to claim Continuous Medical Education credit and Maintenance of Certification (MOC).

The Multidisciplinary Cancer Management Course (MCMC) trains physicians and other health workers in LMICs on the care of the cancer patient with a multidisciplinary emphasis. Each course focuses on the management of the most prevalent cancers in each region, covering the roles of each member of the care team through an interactive combination of lectures, discussions, and case presentations. The LMIC collaborating organization plays a key role in defining training goals, customizing training content to the particular practice of the LMIC, and equipping a faculty that is local with what is needed to deliver the courses. A 'Train the Trainer' has been added to the MCMC curriculum to increase the quantity and quality of trainers in the LMIC by teaching a select group of trainers concepts in adult learning and best practices in course implementation

Meanwhile, the ICTWs support cancer research in LMICs by developing research skills among early-career researchers with topics covering:

- Research ethics.
- Best practices in implementing clinical trials.
- Clinical study methodologies.
- Statistics for investigators.
- Regulatory issues.

The Cancer Control in Primary Care course provides primary healthcare providers with practical and specific knowledge that can be put into daily practice. Topics covered in the course include: cancer prevention and awareness, health communication, local resources, and early detection and referral networks. At the other end, the international palliative care workshops teach topics focused on pain assessment, symptom management, and communication skills.

In addition to the above courses, ASCO may endorse an education program of another organization. Such an endorsement conveys that ASCO grants permission to the organization to use the ASCO logo on the program brochure and other program-related material. The educational program, however, is developed primarily by local or regional organizations, and then reviewed and approved by ASCO's International Affairs Committee. Furthermore, ASCO regularly organizes educational meetings and workshops bringing together experts in the field in small, intensive-learning settings to provide attendees with in-depth, case-based training. The ever-expanding roster of workshops and training programs help those in the oncology community stay current, provide the highest quality care to patients, and grow professionally in the fast-paced field of oncology.

2.6.2 Supporting Health Volunteers Overseas

The ASCO's support of Health Volunteers Overseas (HVO), an international medical education organization, provides an opportunity to strengthen cancer care in medical centers in low-resource countries. The program started in 2008, to create a program to pair ASCO's member oncologists with colleagues at medical centers in LMICs that serve as their nations' major cancer referral hospitals. The aim of the 'International Cancer Corps' (ICC) is to exchange medical expertise, develop training programs, and build long-term, supportive relationships between ASCO, these vital medical institutions, and the clinicians who practice there.

By volunteering for HVO's education and training programs, oncology professionals can share their medical expertise and build long-term, supportive relationships with clinicians in these countries. HVO is dedicated to improving the availability and quality of healthcare through the education, training, and professional development of the health workforce in resource-scarce countries.

Volunteers must be appropriately trained and credentialed medical professionals who specialize in oncology. This includes physicians (medical, radiation, surgical oncology, among other specialists), laboratory professionals, and nurses. Final year oncology fellows are accepted if paired with an experienced volunteer. Some HVO Education and Training Sites are in Vietnam, Honduras, Bhutan, and more recently Nepal. The program is active in more than 40 hospitals in 25 countries, with HVO-affiliated medical volunteers training, mentoring, and providing critical professional support to healthcare providers.

2.6.3 ASCO's IDEA program

ASCO's International Development and Education Award (IDEA) is designed to support the professional development of young oncologists from LMICs who can be effective or transformative clinical leaders driving advances in cancer care, research, and education, in their organizations, nationally, regionally, and even across continents in a sustainable way. The crux of the IDEA program is the formation of ASCO member mentor–mentee pairs, with mentees selected through a highly competitive application process. Awardees are carefully matched with a senior ASCO member mentor on the basis of shared clinical and research interests. They attend ASCO's annual meeting and then can participate visit their mentor's institution in the USA or Canada. The award also comes with three years of complimentary ASCO membership, including free subscription to the *Journal of Clinical Oncology*. The crucial component is, however, the following mentoring relationship after the mentee returns to their LMIC.

Hundreds of LMIC participants from over 40 countries have benefitted from this program [35]. IDEA alumni have taken up leadership positions on ASCO committees, received fellowships and other research opportunities, and have pursued longer-term collaborations with their mentors. IDEA alumni share the information and new skills they learned with 50 colleagues, on average, in their LMIC and have helped organize ASCO trainings and other activities in their LMIC. Some have also taken leadership positions in their local or regional societies, even creating oncology societies, in areas where none existed before.

The IDEA program has also now built on their progress an IDEA Palliative Care (IDEA-PC), program to provide support to oncologists who are interested in palliative medicine. Another program is ASCO's Long-term International Fellowship (LIFe), which supports early-career oncologists in LMICs to advance their professional development via deeper relationships with mentors in the USA or Canada. The LIFe program provides funding to support a year-long fellowship, with fellows receiving valuable training and experience, which can be leveraged to effect change in cancer care in their home LMIC. ASCO is apparently committed to continuing to grow these global oncology programs given the apparent impact they are having. More on these ASCO initiatives will be highlighted at the 2017 Harvard Global Health Catalyst summit and in the resulting proceedings.

2.6.4 Global oncology e-learning platforms

Table 2.6 includes a list of some global oncology e-learning platforms.

Table 2.6. Global oncology e-learning platforms.

E-learning platform	Website	Content description
AORTIC: African Organization for Research and Training in Cancer	www.AORTIC-edu.org	All oncology areas.
Paediatric Oncology International Network for Training and Education	www.cancerpointe.com	Promoting global childhood cancer education. Database lists >70 unique training opportunities for healthcare workers in resource-limited settings.
Oncology Education	http://www.oncologyeducation.com	All oncology areas.
International Atomic Energy Agency's VUCCnet	http://cancer.iaea.org/vuccnet.asp	Enables medical professionals at all levels to gain easy access to high-quality training courses to upgrade their skills, without taking time away from work.
eCancer Education	http://ecancer.org/education/education	Free e-learning for any oncology professionals.
e-Oncologia	http://www.e-oncologia.org	All oncology areas.
ASCO University	http://university.asco.org	Life-long continuous learning in oncology.

References

[1] International Agency for Research on Cancer (GLOBOCAN) 2012 *Estimated Cancer Incidence, Mortality, and Prevalence Worldwide in 2012* http://globocan.iarc.fr/Pages/fact_sheets_population.aspx Accessed January 15, 2017

[2] Farmer P, Frenk J and Knaul F M *et al* 2010 Expansion of cancer care and control in countries of low and middle income: a call to action *Lancet* **376** 1186–93
[3] World Health Organization 2016 *Global Strategy on Human Resources for Health: Workforce 2030* (WHO)
[4] Chen L, Evans D and Evans T *et al* 2006 Working together for health. *The World Health Report 2006* www.who.int/whr/2006/whr06_en.pdf Accessed January 16, 2017
[5] Anyangwe S C E and Mtonga C 2007 Inequities in the global health workforce: the greatest impediment to health in sub-Saharan Africa *Int. J. Environ. Res. Public Health* **4** 93–100
[6] Seed Global Health 2017 http://seedglobalhealth.org/ Accessed January 16, 2017
[7] Kerry V B 2012 *Global Health Service Partnership: A Model for Global Health.* www.medscape.com/viewarticle/773798_1 Accessed January 17, 2017
[8] World Bank 2017 *Physicians (per 1000 people): Data* http://data.worldbank.org/indicator/SH.MED.PHYS.ZS Accessed January 20, 2017
[9] World Bank 2017 *Nurses and midwives (per 1000 people): Data* http://data.worldbank.org/indicator/SH.MED.NUMW.P3 Accessed January 20, 2017
[10] Dodani S and La Porte R E 2005 Brain drain from developing countries: how can brain drain be converted into wisdom gain? *J. R. Soc. Med.* **98** 487–91
[11] Kuehn B M 2007 Global shortage of health workers, brain drain stress developing countries *JAMA* **298** 1853–5
[12] Mills E J *et al* 2011 The financial cost of doctors emigrating from sub-Saharan Africa: human capital analysis *Br. Med. J.* **343** d7031
[13] Kerry V B and Mullan F 2014 Global health service partnership: building health professional leadership *Lancet* **383** 1688–91
[14] Bradford Kerry V, Auld S and Farmer P 2010 An international service corps for health—an unconventional prescription for diplomacy *N. Engl. J. Med.* **363** 1199–201
[15] The White House 1961 *Executive Order 10924: Establishment of the Peace Corps (1961)* www.ourdocuments.gov/doc.php?flash=true&doc=92 Accessed January 17, 2017
[16] US Congress 1979 *S. 1424—96th Congress (1979–1980): International Health Act of 1979*
[17] Institute of Medicine 2005 *Healers Abroad: Americans Responding to the Human Resource Crisis in HIV/AIDS* (Washington, DC: National Academies Press)
[18] Mullan F M W 2007 Responding to the global HIV/AIDS crisis *JAMA* **297** 744
[19] Kaplan L 2015 Building healthcare capacity: The Global Health Service Partnership *The Nursing Practitioner* **40** 14–6
[20] Peace Corps Worldwide 2016 *Concept paper for the Peace Corps Global Health Service Partnership* http://peacecorpsworldwide.org/concept-paper-for-the-peace-corps-global-health-service-partnership. Accessed January 17, 2017
[21] Irabor O C, Kerry V, Matton J and Ngwa W 2017 Leveraging the GHSP model for workforce development in global radiation oncology *J. Glob. Oncol.* in press
[22] Global Health Collaborative Uganda Who We Are http://ghcuganda.org/about-us. Accessed January 18, 2017
[23] Passel J S and Cohn D 2008 *US Population Projections: 2005–2050* (Washington DC: Pew Research Center) www.pewsocialtrends.org/2008/02/11/us-population-projections-2005-2050/ Accessed January 18, 2017
[24] Banks J A 2004 Teaching for social justice, diversity, and citizenship in a global world *Ed. Forum.* **68** 289–98
[25] Banks J A 2009 Human rights, diversity, and citizenship education *Ed. Forum.* **73** 100–10

[26] Banks J A (ed) 2004 *Multicultural Education in Global Perspectives: Policy and Institutionalization* (San Francisco, CA: Jossey Bass)

[27] Eav S, Schraub S, Dufou P, Taisant D and Bunda C R P 2012 Oncology in Cambodia *Oncology* **82** 269–74

[28] ASTRO 2013 Global health, members' outreach efforts aid international health care ASTRO News 16 www.astro.org/uploadedFiles/_MAIN_SITE/News_and_Publications/Magazine_(ASTROnews)/Volumes/Summer2013.pdf Accessed June 20, 2017

[29] Ngwa N 2016 *Emerging Models for Global Health in Radiation Oncology* (Bristol: IOP Publishing)

[30] Dittrich C *et al* 2016 ESMO/ASCO recommendations for a global curriculum (GC) in medical oncology *Ann. Oncol.* **27** 1378–81

[31] Dittrich C *et al* 2017 Global curriculum edition 2016: European Society for Medical Oncology/American Society of Clinical Oncology recommendations for training in medical oncology *J. Clin. Oncol.* **35** 254–5

[32] IAEA Syllabus for the Education and Training of Radiation Oncologists. www-pub.iaea.org/MTCD/Publications/PDF/TCS-36_web.pdf Accessed June 20, 2017

[33] Grover S, Chadha M, Rengan R, Williams T R, Morris Z S, Morgan D A, Tripuraneni P, Hu K and Viswanathan A N 2015 Education and training needs in radiation oncology in India: opportunities for Indo–US collaborations *Int. J. Radiat. Oncol.* **93** 957–60

[34] Chen F M, Bauchner H and Burstin H 2004 A call for outcomes research in medical education *Acad. Med.* **79** 955–60 http://www.ncbi.nlm.nih.gov/pubmed/15383351

[35] Pyle D and Daly N 2013 ASCO and the conquer cancer foundation: a global oncology community sharing knowledge to improve patient care *Cancer Control* 147–50

IOP Publishing

Global Oncology
Harvard Global Health Catalyst summit lecture notes
Wilfred Ngwa and Paul Nguyen

Chapter 3

Global oncology research

John Flanigan, Wilfred Ngwa and Jonathan P Celli

3.1 Funding for global oncology research

Lecture by Dr John Flanigan (National Cancer Institute Center for Global Health).

3.1.1 Introduction

The National Cancer Institute (NCI) coordinates the National Cancer Program, which conducts and supports research, training, health information dissemination, and other programs with respect to the cause, diagnosis, prevention, and treatment of cancer, rehabilitation from cancer, and the continuing care of cancer patients and the families of cancer patients. The NCI provides research grants and cooperative agreements to coordinate and support research projects conducted by universities, hospitals, research foundations, and businesses throughout the United States and abroad. NCI also supports education and training in fundamental sciences and clinical disciplines for participation in basic and clinical research programs and treatment programs relating to cancer through career awards, training grants, and fellowships.

Present statics shows that 80% of worldwide non-communicable disease (NCD)—basically cardiovascular diseases, cancers, diabetes and chronic lung diseases—mortality occurs in low and middle income countries (LMICs). Out of 12.7 million of cancer diagnoses per year, more than half are found in LMICs. This implies 2/3 of cancer deaths take place in LMICs with 15% of the world's annual deaths occurring only due to cancer. There are more cancer deaths in LMICs than adding together the deaths due to HIV, malaria, and TB (figure 3.1). Unfortunately less than 1% of the gross domestic product (GDP) of LMICs is spent on R&D [1]. It is expected that by 2030 these numbers are going to change for the worse due to population expansion, upward age shift, shift in disease burden, and increasing costs of treatments.

doi:10.1088/978-0-7503-1359-9ch3

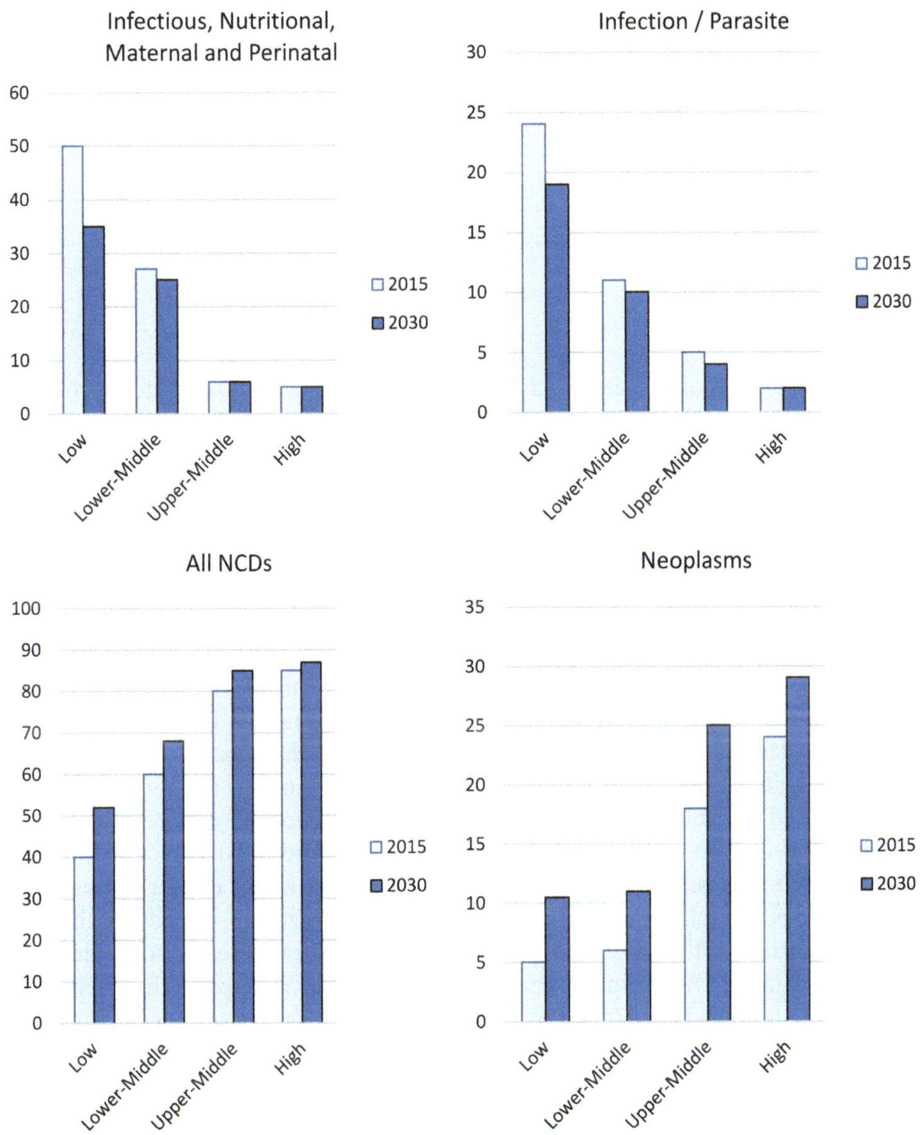

Economy	2015	2030
Low	886 (12.2%)	1,181 (14.3%)
Lower Middle Income	2679 (37%)	3219 (38.9%)
Upper Middle Income	2565 (35.4%)	2696 (32.5%)
High	1118 (15.4%)	1187 (14.3%)

Figure 3.1. Rising burden of cancer and non-communicable diseases. Reproduced with permission from [2]

Table 3.1. The income level of upper, upper-middle, lower-middle, and low income countries. Data from [3].

Income level	Range (in USD)	Countries
High	>$12 746	75
Upper-middle	$4035–12 475	55
Lower-middle	$1026–4035	50
Low	<$1025	34

3.1.2 Challenge of funding

Considering the World Bank Classification system and taking into account 214 countries in terms of economics, table 3.1 shows the income level of upper, upper-middle, lower-middle, and low income countries.

There are three major global funding information platforms: the World RePORT (worldreport.nih.gov), the International Cancer Research Partnership (ICRP), and the Global Oncology Cancer Resource Map. The World RePORT is hosted by the US National Institutes of Health and managed through a steering committee of the agencies providing data. To maintain World RePORT as open-access to the entire research community, in particular those conducting research in LMICs, this effort has been sponsored by the United States National Institutes of Health (NIH), the United Kingdom Medical Research Council (MRC), and the Bill & Melinda Gates Foundation (BMGF), with pledged support from the European Commission (EC), Canadian Institutes of Health Research, and the Wellcome Trust.

Established in 2000, the ICRP is a unique alliance of cancer organizations working together to enhance global collaboration and strategic coordination of research. The aim is to improve access to information about cancer research being conducted and enable cancer organizations to maximize the impact of their independent efforts, for the benefit of researchers and cancer patients worldwide. ICRP includes organizations from Australia, Canada, France, Japan, the Netherlands, United Kingdom, and the United States. The ICRP database contains information on 77 885 grants, totaling over $50 billion in cancer research since 2000 from 110 funding organizations. Researchers can search the ICRP to avoid duplication and identify collaborators.

Meanwhile, the nonprofit Global Oncology Inc. (GO) announced the launch of the Global Cancer Project Map, a novel online resource and virtual information exchange connecting the global cancer community. Developed by GO in collaboration with the NCI Center for Global Health (NIC/CGH), the Map enables worldwide access to cancer projects and expertise, improving cancer practices and patient outcomes, particularly in low-resource settings.

According to the World RePORT for funded projects for different countries, the projects funded are greater in number for low income countries than upper/upper-middle countries. Table 3.2 highlights the results. South Africa skews the list as an upper-middle income country and Equatorial Guinea is seen as a high income state. The World RePORT dataset is currently limited to sub-Saharan Africa

Table 3.2. Funded projects, World RePORT 2013.

Economy	Population	Projects	Projects/million
High	722 254	0	0.00
Upper-middle	26 537 698	94	3.54
Lower-middle	290 247 972	430	1.48
Low	535 405 887	1544	2.88

3.1.3 Cancer research training

The cancer training and career development opportunities offered by NCI cover a broad spectrum of disciplines for individuals at career stages ranging from high school students, graduate students, scientists, clinicians, and healthcare professionals. A number of short course cancer research education programs are ongoing.

One of them is the NCI Summer Curriculum in Cancer Prevention, which runs for about five weeks and involves around 25–45 LMIC participants. There is no fee with some support. Another example is the International Agency for Research on Cancer (IARC) Summer School conducted in Lyon to stimulate research in cancer epidemiology and cancer prevention by improving scientific knowledge and developing skills among researchers worldwide. There are also numerous Grant Writing Workshops by the NCI/CGH, other NIH ICs, WHO/PAHO, WHO/AFRO, the Wellcome Trust, CDC, USAID, IARC, UICC, SAMRC, the Ministry of Health, Colombia, CARPHA, etc. There are also International Clinical Trial Workshops organized by ASCO and the NCI/CGH.

Clinical Trial Development Workshops are also organized by ASCO and AACR. According to Vailworkshop.org [4], these intensive workshops have been designed to increase the reliability and effectiveness of clinical trials by:

- 'Introducing clinical fellows and junior faculty in any oncology subspecialty to the principles of good clinical trial design. This Workshop gives them the tools they need to conduct clinical trials that will yield clear results and have the potential to impact patient care.
- Exposing early-career clinical scientists to the full spectrum of challenges in clinical research—from surgery, radiotherapy, conventional and investigational agents, multidisciplinary treatment regimens, multimodality and combination treatments, and the integration of biomarkers in clinical trials. Workshop faculty seek to inspire participants to devote all or a portion of their future careers to some aspect of clinical research.
- Developing a cadre of well-trained, experienced clinical researchers whose expertise will foster better clinical trial design. Such expertise will thereby hasten the introduction of improved approaches for cancer therapy and prevention into everyday medical practice and patient care.'

In addition to short research training courses, there are a number of LMIC graduate research and postdoctoral fellowships offered by the NCI, and also other organizations such as IRDC (Canada), Fogarty International Center (FIC), Institute Pasteur, MSCA (Europe), INSERM (France), etc. Furthermore, there are career development fellowships for LMIC investigators available abroad from organizations such as ASCO, ESMO, World Bank, and UICC. The Fogarty awards include the Global Health Initiative for New Foreign Investigators, Global Health Research and Training eCapacity, Informatics Training for Health Professionals, and other institutional-level programs.

For health research and development, many organizations offer programs across the world including: The Global Health Research Institute and IDRC in Canada; The European Research Council; the Swedish International Development and Cooperation Agency (SIDA); the UK Medical Research Council/DFID; the US Agency for International Development (USAID); the PEER Program: NSF, USAID, NIH/NCI; the Bill & Melinda Gates Foundation; and the Wellcome Trust.

We have two million cancers per year worldwide due to infectious etiologies. There are various LMIC funding opportunities in the field of infectious disease. These include the European Clinical Trials Partnership (for sub-Saharan Africa only), WHO, the Special Program for Research and Training in Tropical Diseases (TDR), and the Global Fund to Fight AIDS, Tuberculosis, and Malaria. There are also the organizations Pink Ribbon/Red Ribbon and Rwanda: Human Resources for Health. There are also LMIC cancer-specific funding opportunities including: the US NCI, The French National Cancer Institute, American Cancer Society, Cancer Research UK, Susan Komen Foundation, World Cancer Research Foundation, and the American Association for Cancer Research.

3.1.4 The National Institute of Health (NIH): annual funding

The mission of the United States NIH is to seek fundamental knowledge about the nature and behavior of living systems and the application of that knowledge to enhance health, lengthen life, and reduce illness and disability. About $30.1 billion (figure 3.2 and 3.3), more than 80% of the NIH's funding, is awarded through almost

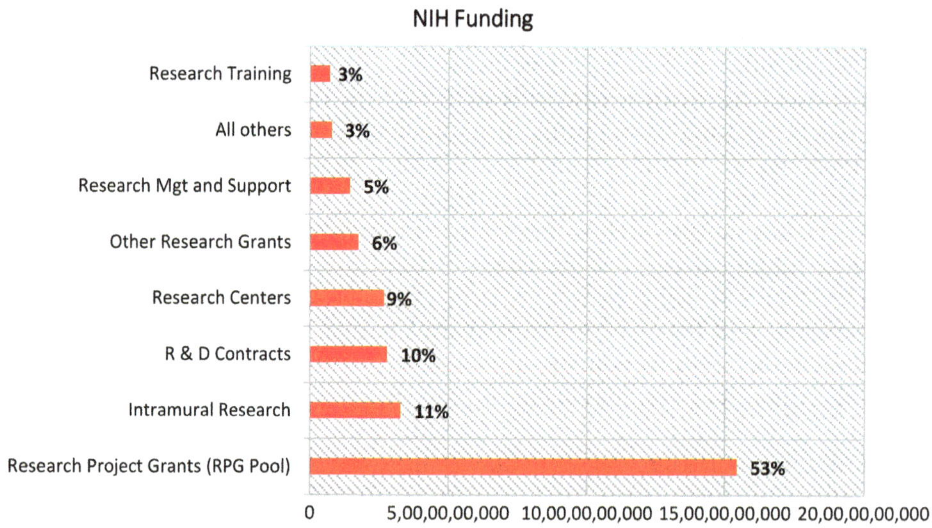

Figure 3.2. NIH funding. Reproduced with permission from [5].

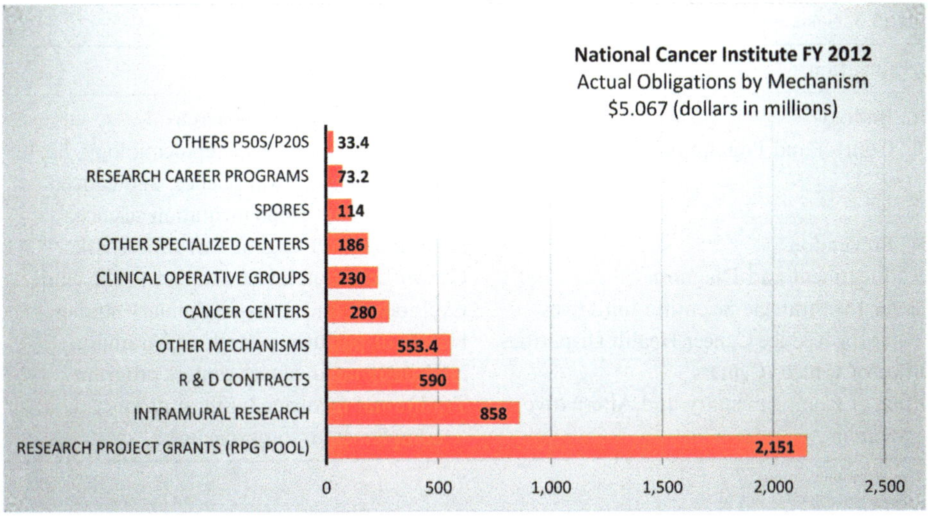

Figure 3.3. NCI funding portfolio. Reproduced with permission from [5].

Foreigmts of U.S. Domestic Research Grants and Contracts in FY2013

(This textramural grants and contracts only; intramural projects are excluded.)

	Funding Mechanism																
Country	D43	F30	F31	F32	K01	K05	K07	K23	N02	R01	R03	R21	R25	R37	U01	U24	UM1
Argentina					1					1						1	
Bangladesh										3							
Belarus									1								
Benin										1							
Brazil										3			1		1	1	
Cameroon	1									1							
China							1			17	3			1	2	2	1
Columbia										1						1	
Dominican Rep										1							
Egypt										3						1	
Honduras											1						
Hungary																2	
India				1		1				4	1					1	

* Partial list for legibility.

Figure 3.4. NCI funding portfolio for LMICs.

50 000 competitive grants to more than 300 000 researchers at more than 2500 universities, medical schools, and other research institutions in every state and around the world. Of this the NCI spends ~5 billion on research grants.

Direct grants by NCI to LMICs are rare, as highlighted by figure 3.4. There are NCI grants that are eligible to have foreign components, ranging in the millions of

Table 3.3. Some NCI funding organizations.

Organization	Mission
DC Biology	Basic cancer biology research.
DC Control and Population Science	Research in surveillance, epidemiology, health services, behavioral science, and cancer survivorship. Implementation science.
DC Prevention	Determination/mitigation of cancer risk.
DC Treatment and Diagnosis	Cancer detection and treatment to the clinic.
Center for Strategic Scientific Initiatives	Exploratory and trans-disciplinary studies.
Center for Reduce Cancer Health Disparities	Health disparities research and training.
Office of Cancer Centers	NCI-designated cancer centers program.
Office of Complementary and Alternative Medicine	Traditional medicine, natural product discovery, complementary approaches.

dollars, for various countries such as Argentina, Bangladesh, Belarus, Benin, Brazil, Cameroon, China, Colombia, the Dominican Republic, Egypt, Honduras, Hungary, and India, to name a few. There are also grants available for LMIC clinical treatment trials from the NCI.

There are also other extramural funding opportunities by NCI that are managed by different organizations. These are highlighted in table 3.3.

In 2011, the National Cancer Institute (NCI) established the Center for Global Health (CGH) to help reduce the global burden of cancer. CGH develops initiatives and collaborates with other NCI divisions, NCI-designated cancer centers, and countries to support cancer control planning build capacity, and support cancer research and cancer research networks in LMICs. Funding opportunities have included: a short-term (six month) scientist (MD or PhD) exchange program to and from LMICs; low-cost technology for health research in LMICs, supporting development of low-cost tech for detection, diagnosis, and treatment; and the BIG Cat program administered via AORTIC (D43 mechanism) with pilot funding of up to $25k for Africa only. Table 3.4 highlights some of the opportunities provided by Fogarty International Center (FIC).

FIC also provides grants for US investigators (table 3.5). These are designed to provide experiences in LMICs. These include the International Research Scientist Development Award for US citizens with a doctoral-level degree in a research or health-related field. This comes with a condition that the awardee must spend at least 50% of their time in an LMIC institution and have both LMIC- and US-based mentors. There is also the Fulbright-Fogarty Fellows in Public Health award. This is limited to medical and graduate students who are US citizens to conduct research projects in an eligible LMIC. Meanwhile the Fulbright-Fogarty Scholars in Public Health award is limited to postdoctoral students in public health research who are US citizens and who will conduct research at a Fogarty-affiliated site in a specific LMIC.

Table 3.4. FIC opportunities for LMICs.

Organization	Mission
International Cooperative Biodiversity Groups	Biodiversity/natural product discovery; support for sustainable natural resource utilization.
Chronic, NCDs and Disorders Across the Lifespan: FIC International Training Award	Strengthen research capacity for NCDs; encourage implementation of evidence-based public health measures appropriate for locale.
Global Health Research and Training eCapacity Initiative	Award supports integration of ICT by previous awardees.
Informatics Training for Global Health	Up to 5 yrs support for US/LMIC collaborators to integrate informatics.
Global Health Initiative for New Investigators	Career development grant for LMIC investigators who have returned to their home country.
FIC International Research Collaboration Award	Co-support from multiple ICs: benefits both US and LMIC collaborators.
International Research Ethics Education and Curriculum Dev.	Funds development of masters-level curriculum for research institutions in LMICs
Framework Programs for Global Health Innovations (FRAME Innovation)	Support for both US and LMIC for interdisciplinary, postdoctoral research training directed towards encouraging innovation in health-related products, processes and policies.
International Tobacco and Health Research and Capacity Building Program	For LMIC institutions promoting trans-disciplinary research to decrease tobacco morbidity/mortality.
Medical Partnership Initiative (MEPI)	Available only to LMIC institutions that have previously received support from PEPFAR and PEPFAR partners to develop and improve medical education

Table 3.5. FIC grants for USA investigators.

Organization	Mission
International Research Scientist Development Award	Applicants must be U.S. citizens with a doctoral-level degree in a research or health-related field. The awardee must spend at least 50% time in an LMIC institution and have both LMIC and U.S.-based mentors.
Fulbright-Fogarty Fellows in Public Health	This is limited to medical and graduate students who are U.S. citizens and who will conduct research projects in an eligible LMIC.
Fulbright-Fogarty Scholars in Public Health	This is limited to postdoctoral students in public health research who are U.S. citizens and who will conduct research at a Fogarty-affiliated site in a specific LMIC.

3.2. Information and communication technology powered approaches for global radiation oncology research

Lecture notes by Wilfred Ngwa.

3.2.1. Introduction

In recent publications [6–9], we have highlighted the tremendous potential of information and communication technologies (ICTs) in catalyzing high impact international collaborations in global radiation oncology. Here ICTs are considered to be technologies used in the transmission, manipulation, and storage of data by electronic means, including the internet, mobile phone systems, broadcast radio, TV systems, and so forth. In a lecture by Professor Janaki Moni during the Global Health Catalyst (GHC) summit, the potential role of the ICT-powered Quality Assurance Review Center (QARC) platform [6] in global radiation oncology research was presented and discussed.

In 1980, the QARC was founded to provide radiation therapy quality assurance (QA) services to the National Cancer Cooperative Groups funded by the National Cancer Institute (NCI). Over the next three decades QARC added diagnostic imaging data management and review facilitation to its portfolio of services. In November 2011 the NCI announced the transition of the Cooperative Group program to a new National Clinical Trials Network (NCTN). In 2013, a new model for imaging and radiation therapy QA in the NCTN of the NCI was reported [10, 11]. In the new model QARC has joined with five other legacy QA centers to form a new organization known as IROC (Imaging and Radiation Oncology Core Cooperative) to serve the NCTN. Under the IROC umbrella these six highly experienced QA centers will provide an integrated program with standardized services to the entire NCTN. Within the NCTN, QARC is now IROC RI and will continue to provide services to the NCI as it has for over three decades.

The QARC mission is to provide superior services in support of cancer clinical trials to improve the standards of care in the management of cancer by advancing the quality of clinical trials medicine. Typical radiotherapy QARC programs/services include: protocol development, site credentialing and performance, data acquisition, data management, data archiving, case evaluation and feedback to clinical trial investigators, and secondary research projects.

The ICT-powered QARC has two integrated components: the MAX and the CERR. The MAX (figure 3.5) is a relational database and image management system. It maintains records on patients enrolled in clinical trials, maintains information on over 1500 participating institutions, contains a patient electronic imaging archive (PEI), and is fully 21 Code of Federal Regulations ('CFR') Part 11 compliant in protecting patient privacy [6].

Meanwhile the Computational Environment for Radiotherapy Research (CERR) [12] component was developed by Deasy *et al* as a software integration environment to combine treatment planning software written in multiple languages (MATLAB, FORTRAN, C/C++, JAVA, etc), together with treatment plan information

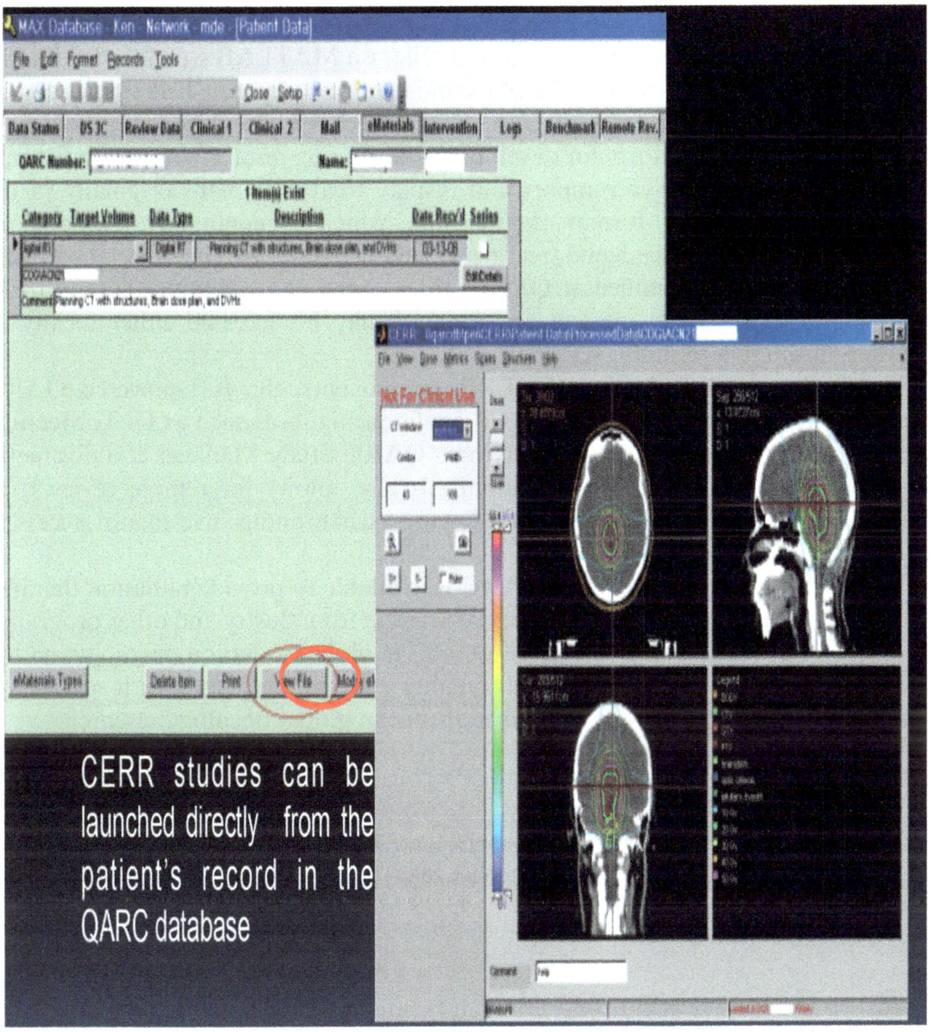

Figure 3.5. MAX database integrated in the ICT-powered QARC platform. Reproduced with permission from [11]

(computed tomography scans, outlined structures, dose distributions, digital films, etc). It also provides the ability to extract treatment plans from disparate planning systems using the widely available AAPM/RTOG archiving mechanism, and it provides a convenient and powerful tool for sharing and reproducing treatment planning results. CERR's functional components include: (1) an import program which converts the widely available AAPM/RTOG treatment planning format into a MATLAB cell-array data object, facilitating manipulation; (2) viewers which display axial, coronal, and sagittal computed tomography images, structure contours, digital films, and isodose lines or dose colorwash; (3) a suite of contouring tools to edit and/or create anatomical structures; (4) dose–volume and dose–surface histogram calculation and display tools; and (5) various predefined commands. The code is relatively self-describing, because it relies on MATLAB structure field name definitions based on the AAPM/RTOG standard. New structure field names can be added dynamically or permanently. In short, CERR (pronounced 'sir') provides a convenient software platform for developing and sharing results in radiation therapy treatment planning and can import and display treatment plans originally in the AAPM/RTOG archive format (figure 3.6), which is commonly available in commercial and many academic treatment planning systems. The original software has been extensively modified at QARC. Files containing radiation therapy treatment plans are linked to patient records and may be accessed either locally or remotely through a terminal server.

In addition to the MAX and CERR components, the ICT-powered QARC allows for remote reviews via web-based conferencing tools such as GoToMeeting, WebEx etc. This has the benefit of having a QARC Study Manager and dosimetry staff available synchronously for support. It also allows for remote reviews via remote access. This has the benefit of allowing asynchronous investigator access to his/her cases at their convenience.

In addition to serving the NCI, QARC is available to provide radiation therapy, diagnostic imaging, and data management services for industry and other programs. Here we propose extending the use of QARC in global radiation oncology, with a vision to eventually establish regional Quality Assurance Centers with services to LMIC institutions not only in clinical trials but in global oncology research.

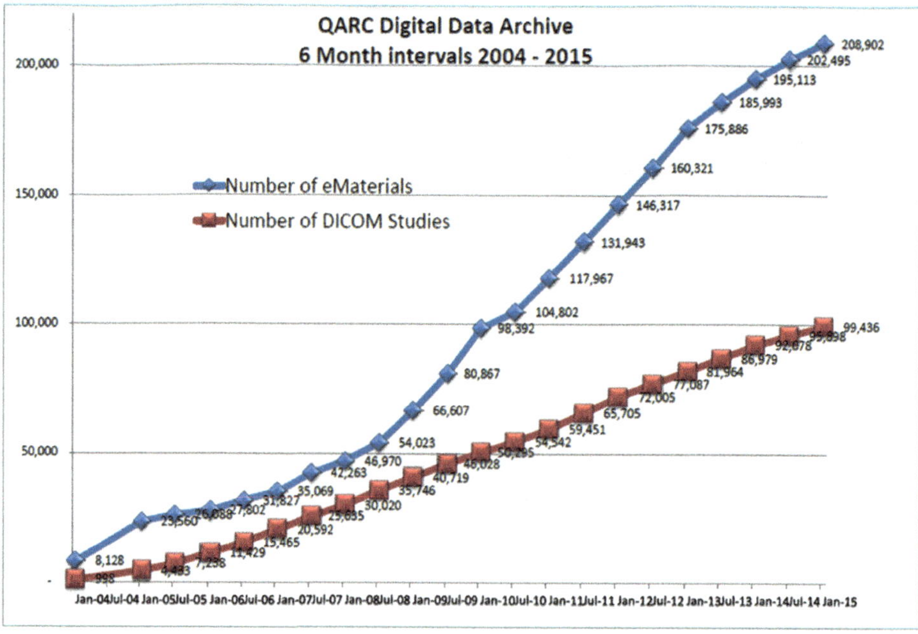

Figure 3.6. Sample data from the QARC digital data archive. Reproduced with permission from [11]

3.2.2 Global oncology research powered by the QARC

QARC could be employed for global oncology research in a number of ways. These include the use of QARC in facilitating international 'chart rounds', which have been identified as valuable in cancer care and continuous education. Chart rounds may also benefit the training of high income country (HIC) radiation oncology health professionals or residents as these can be highly educational. In the course of doing this QARC could be used to maintain a registry of patients discussed. Furthermore, QARC could be used to connect other arrays, such as genetic or pathology information, to appropriate research databases.

According to the NCI, many of the same population groups that experience cancer health disparities are also significantly underrepresented in cancer clinical trials. One of the ways to close the cancer divide, eliminating disparities, is to include minorities, or populations from disparate backgrounds and resource-poor settings in clinical trials. Given the growing global burden of cancer, major global disparities, and substantive interest by radiation oncology health professionals in African LMICs to participate in multi-center clinical trials, the QARC platform is clearly an excellent system to employ for multi-center clinical trials involving LMIC institutions.

A companion to NCI's NCTN, the NCI Community Oncology Research Program (NCORP) supports community-based clinical trials and cancer care delivery research. These community-based studies are helping to address cancer health disparities by increasing participation by minorities and patients from underserved populations in clinical cancer research. In a recent study [11], they found that cancer patients who live on less than $50 000 a year take part in clinical trials at a rate one-third lower than those who make more annually. Because clinical trials often provide the most cutting edge—if still unproven—treatments, the finding is a new example of how income disparities translate to unequal access to medical care. This disparity is even worse for LMICs, e.g. in Africa, and is therefore a major area that needs to be addressed in efforts to close the cancer divide. Enrolling LMIC patients would be a benefit for both researchers and for patients. The research benefits because trials can be done more quickly with increased participation and they would be more representative. For patients, clinical trials are a vital resource, so there should not be a disparity depending on your income. LMIC investigators in Africa are particularly motivated to participate in clinical trials given the growing burden of cancer and the fact that most cancer patients in Africa often present with advanced metastatic disease and could greatly benefit from clinical trials including ones investigating new low-cost approaches for cancer treatment.

Clinical trials are the only accepted scientific method to test if a new treatment is safe and effective in humans. In addition to new therapies, some trials test giving already approved treatments at lower doses, on different schedules or in new combinations, which could improve care. In radiation oncology, hypofractionation has been proposed as a more effective approach to increase access to treatment for patients in LMICs [3]. This appears to be one initial multi-center clinical trial, even just amongst LMIC institutions, that could be conducted leveraging the QARC system. Combination treatments and new low-cost approaches for radiotherapy that can benefit many cancer patients in LMICs could also benefit from the use of QARC and associated services.

In summary, QARC provides an ICT-powered platform that could go a long way in facilitating collaborations in cancer research and education, advancing efforts to close the cancer divide, and thus eliminate global cancer disparities.

3.3 Low-cost technologies for global oncology

3.3.1 Photodynamic therapy for oral cancer: low-cost enabling technology for global health

Lecture by Professor Jonathan P Celli.

3.3.1.1 Introduction

It is estimated that oral cancer claims one life every six hours in India alone. This is partly caused by widespread chewing of carcinogenic tobacco/betel nut/acacia extract. Oral cancer accounts for approximately 30% of the reported cancer cases in India. This includes over 80 000+ new cases/year [13]. Surgery and radiotherapy are inaccessible to many patients and even when curative therapy is possible, surgery/radiotherapy in the oral cavity often impairs quality of life (dry mouth, chewing, swallowing, speaking, etc). There is urgent need for effective, yet low-cost, treatment and imaging in sites with limited medical infrastructure. Here we briefly describe ongoing collaborative work at the University of Massachusetts Boston and the Wellman Center for Photomedicine, Massachusetts General Hospital, to develop low-cost enabling technologies for photodynamic therapy (PDT) treatment of oral lesions in an effort to address this unmet clinical need in India.

PDT is a light-based therapeutic modality with several inherent features that suggest its promise for treatment of oral cancers in India and other low and middle income (LMIC) settings [14, 15]. In PDT, a photosensitizing agent or precursor is first administered and will accumulate somewhat preferentially in malignant tissues [15]. These agents are non-toxic in the absence of light, but can impart cytotoxicity by photochemical reactions involving singlet oxygen and other products of photochemical reactions. After sufficient time for uptake and tumor localization the photosensitized malignant tissue is activated by light, usually using red or near-infrared wavelengths. Although medical lasers may be costly in resource-limited settings, PDT light sources can also be constructed using low-cost LEDs, and built to operate on battery power to be adapted for use in remote or rural sites. In addition to therapy, photosensitizing agents virtually all have some fluorescence, allowing high contrast fluorescent imaging of lesions that can be leveraged as a powerful tool for therapeutic guidance and monitoring [15].

3.3.1.2 PDT for oral cancers

Previous clinical results with aminolevulinic acid (ALA) as a photosensitizer precursor (leading to accumulation of the endogenous photosensitizer protoporphyrin IX) for PDT treatment of oral lesions PDT are promising, in particular for thin lesions and oral pre-cancers, with complete epithelial necrosis and excellent healing of mucosa [14]. But adaptations are needed for sustainable global health implementation. Desirable characteristics include: low-cost components, operation with minimal medical infrastructure (no operating room, etc), stable operation without electricity (battery power), devices that are robust/rugged/portable and simple to use with the potential for integration with telemedicine.

A low-cost fiber-coupled, battery operated device for intraoral PDT has been developed (figure 3.7). The device constitutes a fiber coupled to an internal 635 nm LED PDT (optimal PpIX activation). Light of approximately 35–180 mW cm^{-2} irradiance is used, depending on the applicator and lesion size. In contact mode light delivery, e.g. for a typical 100 J cm^{-2} light dose, the treatment can last 10–30 min. The device runs on a rechargeable battery pack (stable output for 1+ hour continuous), or wall power (if available).

For imaging-based guidance of therapy in a setting with limited medical infrastructure the tumor-selective fluorescence contrast provided by PpIX can be imaged using simple adaptations of a standard consumer smartphone. Early results in titanium dioxide tissue phantoms show the ability to resolve clinically relevant PpIX concentrations [14]. The implementation of smartphones as the basis of an imaging platform is also significant given the high extent of smartphone penetration in India, in addition to the potential for integration with telemedicine. The concept of smartphone-based fluorescence imaging for treatment guidance and monitoring is illustrated schematically in figure 3.8.

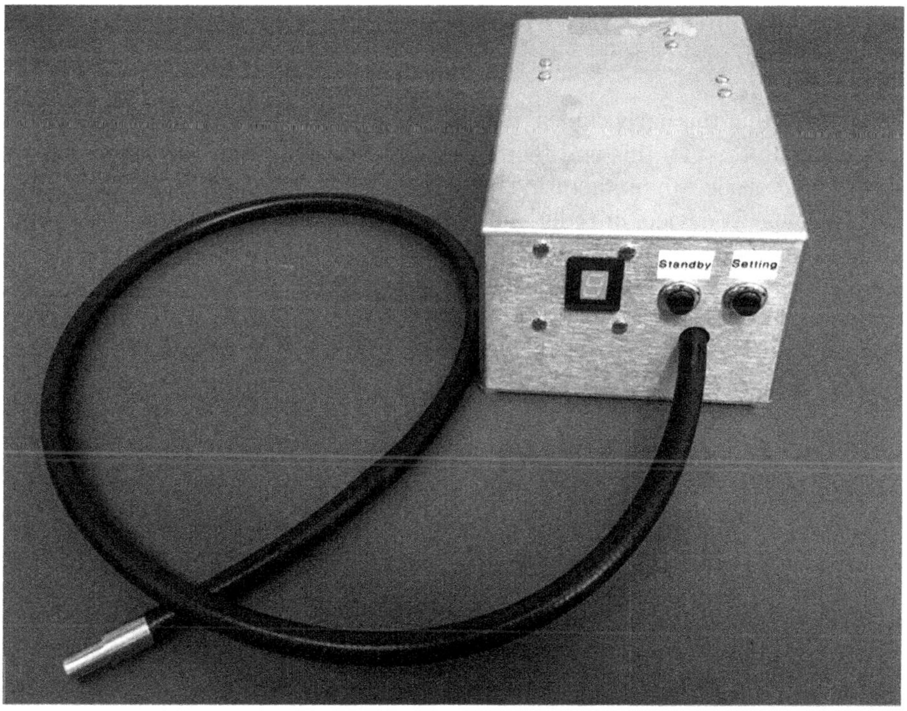

Figure 3.7. A low-cost fiber-coupled, battery operated device for intraoral PDT.

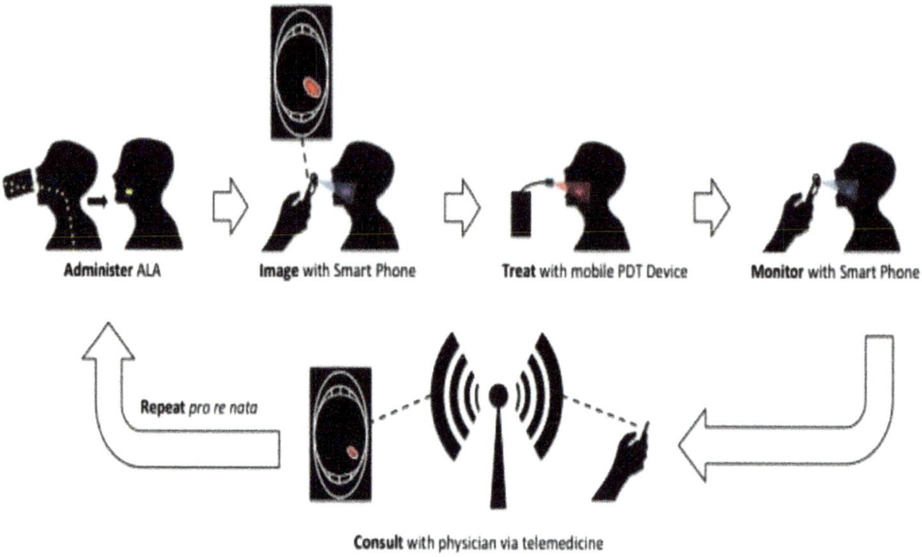

Figure 3.8. Envisioned implementation of image-guided PDT for oral cancers with telemedicine integration. Reproduced with permission from [14]

3.3.1.3 Ongoing developments

The work described here has led to an initial feasibility study at a collaborating LMIC site in Uttar Pradesh, India. Beginning in the spring of 2017, 30 patients are being recruited through Aligarh Muslim University/JN Medical College with early stage (T1N0M0) oral cancers for a feasibility study using low-cost technologies for image-guided PDT.

It is hoped that this early clinical work will lead to robust efforts to establish long-term sustainability. To this end there are efforts to work with the pharmaceutical industry and device manufacturing partners can sustainably commercialize and market a low-cost device, in India and beyond. This work is also being coordinated with training and local outreach in India via collaborations. If successful the technology could be scaled or extended to other LMIC sites with high oral cancer incidence.

3.3.2 Smart radiotherapy biomaterials

By Wilfred Ngwa

Radiotherapy (RT) is employed in the treatment of over 50% of cancer patients either alone or in combination with other treatments such as surgery or chemotherapy [8, 16]. The ultimate goal of RT is to maximize damage to the cancer cells, while minimizing toxicities to healthy tissue. Major advances have been made over the past few decades, as improvements in engineering and computing have enabled RT modalities such as intensity modulated radiotherapy (IMRT), stereotactic ablative radiotherapy (SABR), and image guided radiotherapy (IGRT) to be used in routine clinical practice.

Today, patients undergoing IGRT or brachytherapy routinely have inert RT biomaterials implanted into their tumors. These inert RT biomaterials include fiducial markers, spacers, transponders (beacons), and balloon applicators, engineered to be used in RT treatment of patients with lung, pancreatic, breast, prostate, liver cancers, and other tumors exhibiting motion or deformation during RT [17–25]. Currently the inert RT biomaterials have only one function, which is to ensure geometric accuracy during the treatment, in order to enhance therapeutic efficacy.

With these RT biomaterials already having such unfettered access to the tumor sub-volume, there is strong rationale for upgrading the single function inert biomaterials to multifunctional or 'smart' ones that can deliver additional therapeutic or treatment enhancing benefits [26–31]. In general, biomaterials are materials other than foods or drugs designed for specific medical uses, that interrelate with biological systems [32–34]. Smart biomaterials [35–37] are specifically designed to be sensitive to a specific stimulus, such as tumor micro-environment, temperature, pH, the wavelength or intensity of light, or an electrical or magnetic field, and to then respond in active ways, including changing their structure for drug delivery, radioprotection, priming an immune response, and other functions that could cogently enhance therapy.

In 2010, Cormack *et al* [30] proposed using smart RT biomaterials (SRBs): brachytherapy spacers or fiducials loaded with radiosensitizing drugs that could be activated by the tumor microenvironment, post implantation, to sustainably deliver the radiosensitizing drug directly into the tumor sub-volume. The authors concluded that drug loading of implantable devices routinely used in IGRT provides new opportunities for therapy modulation via biological *in situ* dose painting. Later, Kumar *et al* [27] reported on such brachytherapy spacers for delivery of localized chemoradiotherapy. Their results demonstrated that such spacers with customizable release profiles have potential in improving the combined therapeutic efficacy of chemoradiation therapy.

Other scientists have also been developing the use of high atomic number nanoparticles such as gold nanoparticles (GNPs) instead of drugs, loaded into spacers, fiducial markers, or balloon applicators to boost RT [27, 30, 37, 38]. Combining RT and immunotherapy using such SRBs in treating metastatic disease, with minimal toxicities to healthy tissue, is also being investigated [39]. Major advantages of using SRBs include the fact that programmed sustained *in situ* delivery of drugs or nanoparticles directly into the tumor sub-volume from these biomaterials may overcome physiological barriers allowing direct delivery of sufficiently potent payload into the tumor. With the typical intravenous drug delivery approach, less than 5% of a drug reaches the tumor, while the use of SRBs could enable direct delivery into a tumor. The SRB delivery approach would also significantly minimize any systemic/overlapping toxicities. This takes into account the fact that the nanoparticles, such as GNPs, are relatively non-toxic [40–42], and that controlled *in situ* release of nanoparticles or drugs leads to minimal systemic toxicities [43–45]. Second, SRBs could simply replace currently used inert RT biomaterials and so can be employed at no additional inconvenience to cancer patients. Third, the sustained or controlled release and intra-tumor bio-distribution of payloads from the SRBs can be customized or controlled by varying the design parameters, such as payload concentration, polymer type or weight, nanoparticle size, etc, allowing for optimization to RT schedules and for superior therapeutic efficacy.

Given this rationale and advantages, SRBs represent a promising area of research and development. This could lead to new generation RT biomaterials designed to perform their primary functions as conventional inert SRBs, but also controllably deliver therapy enhancing payloads *in situ*, amongst other potential functions for optimal diagnostic and therapeutic efficacy. More broadly, SRBs may also include functionalized stimulus-responsive nanoparticles that can be targeted and activated to boost RT [27, 46]. Such smart nanomaterials could themselves be incorporated into the traditional RT biomaterials [28]. Targeting the nanoparticles is desirable because once nanoparticles are released into the tumor microenvironment, their uptake and retention in cells is important, as well as functionalization to reach sub-cellular targets such as the nucleus [47] or mitochondrion [48] in order to have maximal effect.

Research and development of SRBs [27–30] is still in its early stages, but there are many lessons that can be learned from previous work on smart biomaterials developed for other *in vivo* applications. Research in this area requires cross-disciplinary collaborations and may even leverage international collaborations given some of the applications being considered.

3.3.2.1 Design and structure of smart radiotherapy biomaterials

Design

A smart biomaterial is designed or structured to perform sensing, and actuation [35, 49]. One design of SRBs is illustrated in figure 3.9. This simple design integrates a

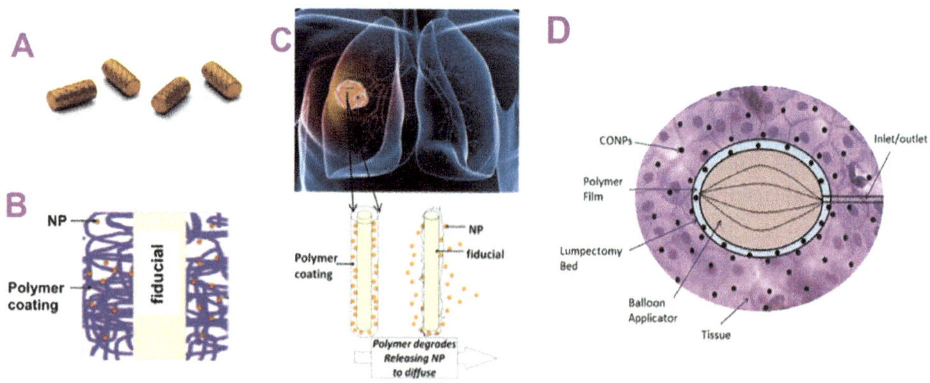

Figure 3.9. (A) Currently used commercially available inert RT biomaterials, e.g. fiducials (CIVCO Medical). (B) One design (not to scale) of an SRB. SRBs could simply replace the inert biomaterials used for (C) IGRT, e.g. for lung cancer, and (D) accelerated partial breast irradiation (loaded here with cerium oxide nanoparticles for selective protecting of healthy breast tissue). Once in place the SRBs can be activated to sustainably release the payload *in situ* directly into the planning target volume. The release and distribution of payload could be customized or optimized to RT schedules as reported in recent studies.

commercially available fiducial marker (figure 3.9(A)) into a smart polymer coating which can sense and actuate or change structure to release a payload incorporated in its polymer matrix (figure 3.9(B)). The choice of smart polymer depends on the nature of the stimulus that would be used to initiate a response. Hitherto studies [27–29, 50] have favored the use of smart synthetic polymers such as poly(l-glycolic acid) (PLGA), and/or natural biological polymers such as chitosan. PLGA is a polymer which is used in a host of Food and Drug Administration (FDA) approved therapeutic devices, owing to its biodegradability and biocompatibility, while chitosan is also widely used in a number of biological applications.

Once in place, the SRB can be activated by a stimulus, e.g. the tumor microenvironment, heat, sound, or electromagnetic waves, to controllably release the payload *in situ*, directly into the tumor (figure 3.9(C)). In an example reported in recent studies [28, 50] it was shown how gold fiducial markers can be coated with nanoporous polymer matrices incorporating nanoparticles. Different polymer types were investigated including the use of PLGA nanoparticles loaded with fluorescent Coumarin-6, serving as a model for a hydrophobic drug in a biodegradable chitosan matrix. A free drug release system consisting of Doxorubicin, a hydrophilic drug, loaded into a non-degradable polymer poly(methyl methacrylate) (PMMA) coating was also demonstrated.

Other designs for SRBs that have been developed include those where, instead of coating commercially available SRBs, a completely new SRB is developed loaded with the payload. This latter approach has the advantage of higher loading capacity. In one example of such a new-design SRB [27, 51], the authors fabricated implantable chemoradiation therapy (INCeRT) spacers loaded with silica nanoparticles (SNPs) containing a drug, to act as a slow-release drug depot for simultaneous localized chemoradiation therapy. The spacers were made of PLGA as the matrix and are physically identical in size to the commercially available brachytherapy spacers (5 mm × 0.8 mm). The silica nanoparticles were conjugated with near-infrared fluorophore Cy7.5 as a model drug. The INCeRT spacers were further doped with an anticancer drug, docetaxel. Studies considering the use of other chemotherapy drugs, such as cisplatin or carboplatin nanoparticles, have also been reported [52–54].

A hybrid of the above design models is also conceivable to program or customize for different release rates. These approaches could also be employed for any RT biomaterials including balloon applicators (figure 3.9(D)). Researchers are considering the coating of such balloon applicators with different nanoparticle types e.g. targeted gold nanoparticles for targeted boosting of dose to residual tumor cells during accelerated partial breast irradiation (APBI) [37] or using cerium oxide nanoparticles to selectively protect healthy breast tissue during the same [38], or intraoperative RT.

Smart nanoparticles for radiotherapy

The potent component of SRBs is the payload, which could be nanoparticles or so-called nano-carriers/drones also carrying a payload. A number of excellent recent review papers have covered the field of nanoparticle-aided RT including: GNPs, gadolinium nanoparticles, hafnium oxide nanoparticles, and so forth [26, 55–61]. The growing consensus remains that one major challenge is how to selectively deliver nanoparticles to cancer cells. Functionalizing nanoparticles is a widely used technique that allows for conjugation of the nanoparticles with targeting ligands, which possess the inherent ability to direct selective binding to cell types or states and, therefore, confer 'smartness' to nanoparticles. Friedman *et al* [62] recently published an article on 'smart targeting of nanoparticles', describing the methods of ligand–nanoparticle functionalization, and a cross-section of various ligand classes used, including small molecules, peptides, antibodies, engineered proteins, or nucleic acid aptamers. PEGylation adds stealth, while multifunctionalization could include imaging moieties for different applications [63–69]. Biomaterials scientists [70] have also developed targeted, biodegradable nano 'drones' to deliver drugs which could be adapted for RT applications. Docetaxel (Dtxl)-encapsulated nanoparticles have been formulated with the biocompatible and biodegradable PLGA-block-poly (ethylene glycol) (PLGA-b-PEG) copolymer and a surface functionalized with RNA aptamers that recognize the extracellular domain of the prostate-specific membrane antigen (PSMA). The approach highlights the potential of employing such nanocarriers to deliver payloads that could also enhance RT [71–96].

For RT, there is also growing consensus that delivery of nanoparticles within the tumor sub-volume is necessary but not sufficient to enhance therapy, and that sub-cellular targeting may be crucial in maximizing therapeutic efficacy. This may be particularly important for high atomic number nanoparticles, such as GNPs, which boost RT by emission of short range photo-/Auger electrons with subcellular range. For example, Burger *et al* [47] developed an approach to enhance the uptake of small nanoparticles functionalized with DNA allowing for strong perinuclear focal accumulation. The authors reported that only the GNPs functionalized with DNA showed a significant radiosensitizing effect ($p = 0.005$) on clonogenic survival using clinically relevant megavolt x-rays. Recently, other third generation (3G) [46] and fourth generation (4G) [26] nanoparticles have been optimized for targeted RT applications functionalized with other moieties such as RGD.

In combination therapy approaches, smart or stimuli-responsive nanocarriers loaded, for example, with chemotherapy drugs or immunoadjuvants, have also been reported [75]. Nanoparticles loaded with immunoadjuvants are particularly attractive, as the use of nanoparticles may allow improved antigen stability and immunogenicity, but also targeted delivery and slow release. A number of nanoparticle vaccines varying in composition, size, shape, and surface properties have been approved for human use and the number of candidates is increasing [75, 76]. However, challenges remain due to a lack of fundamental understanding regarding the *in vivo* behavior of nanoparticles, which could operate as either a delivery system to enhance antigen processing or as an immunostimulant adjuvant to activate or enhance immunity. *In situ* delivery of such nanoparticles or immunoadjuvants to prime the abscopal effect during RT is appealing. In addition to nanoparticles, other nanocarriers such as, micelles, carbon nanotubes, water-soluble polymers, liposomes, and dendrimers have been engineered as agents for targeted delivery to benefit tumor diagnosis and therapy [77–81] and could potentially be adapted for enhancing RT.

Meanwhile, Song and co-authors [82] have reported on smart GNPs designed for photoacoustic imaging, an image contrast agent responsive to the tumor micro-environment. Such nanoparticles could be employed to enhance RT treatment via the photoelectric effect while providing imaging functionality. Wong *et al* [83] have also developed a smart multi-stage biomaterial platform in which 100 nm nanoparticles 'shrink' to 10 nm nanoparticles after they extravasate from leaky regions of the tumor vasculature and are exposed to the tumor microenvironment. In general, nanoparticles able to find a target and release their payload upon a specific stimulus are highly attractive for theranostic applications, particularly in cancer. From this perspective, GNPs stand out as suitable multifunctional platforms for the development of efficient delivery, release, and therapy enhancement systems. However, other nanoparticles are also being considered to serve other desirable functions such as 'Gadolinium nanoparticles designed as smart molecular magnetic resonance imaging contrast agents' [84, 85].

3.3.2.2 Potential applications for smart radiotherapy biomaterials

Despite remarkable advances in the development of RT modalities such as IMRT, SABR, and IGRT, major limitations remain in extending the benefits of RT to many more patients to increase their survival and quality of life. SRBs offer opportunities to address some of these limitations in potential clinical applications as follows.

Dose-painting or radiation boosting. In RT practice, a persisting limitation is obviously that of normal tissue toxicity [97–100]. Clinical studies indicate that radiation boosting or dose-painting leads to a significant increase in survival for cancer patients [100, 101]. For example, it has been reported that every 1 Gy boost in biologically effective dose (BED) could lead to 4% relative improvement in survival [101]. However, current modalities for radiation boosting are critically limited by normal tissue toxicity, compounded by respiratory or intra-/inter-fraction tumor motion [100]. An American medical task group report notes that new treatment strategies that can overcome these limitations, allowing an enhanced dose to the tumor while sparing normal tissue, will significantly improve the balance between complications and cure [100].

Nanoparticle-aided RT, e.g. using GNPs, is emerging as a promising new treatment strategy for overcoming these limitations, to enable substantial radiation boosting with minimal toxicity to neighboring healthy tissue [26]. Such targeted nanoparticle-aided RT with GNPs involves first targeting the tumor cells with GNPs, and then targeting the GNPs during RT to boost RT efficacy. In a study by Hainfeld *et al* [102], the use of GNPs with 250 kVp x-rays/photons produced 86% long-term survival as compared to 20% when radiation was used alone, indicating major therapeutic enhancement due to the GNPs. Our own experimental work has also demonstrated the amplification of damage to tumor cells by GNPs [26, 103, 104]. However, the delivery of sufficiently potent concentrations of GNPs to the tumor to boost RT at clinical beam configurations (e.g. 6 MV) is limited, by physiological barriers, in particular when administered intravenously [26]. These physiological barriers in the tumor vasculature are a problem that is particularly pronounced in cancers such as pancreatic cancer

[105]. The use of SRBs could overcome these limitations and therefore is an active area of research.

Leveraging the abscopal effect. Another intrinsic limitation to RT is that it is generally prescribed for treatment of localized disease. However, in 1953, Mole described the abscopal effect [106], whereby localized RT at one site may lead to regression of metastatic cancer at distant sites, which were not irradiated. This potent effect could extend the use of RT from treating localized disease to treat metastatic or systemic disease. In 2004, Formenti and co-authors originally connected the abscopal effect with mechanisms involving the immune system [107]. More recent studies corroborate these findings that the abscopal effect is mediated by the immune system [108–113]. However, the effect is rare because immune-tolerance mechanisms may hamper the development of therapeutically effective responses [113]. A combination of RT and immunoadjuvants could overcome immune-suppression and lead to vigorous anti-tumor T-cell responses [109, 114]. However, while such combinations of RT and immunoadjuvants are promising, their systemic/overlapping toxicities are a major obstacle reported in many studies [108]. The use of SRBs proffers an innovative approach that would minimize such toxicities, and enable slow/sustained *in situ* delivery of nanoparticles with immunoadjuvants, which is expected to enable greater therapeutic efficacy [44]. Early research and previous work from vaccine studies suggests such an approach could indeed be more effective [108]. Investigations in this area are therefore also ongoing.

SRBs could be activated either by the tumor microenvironment, sound, heat, electromagnetic waves, or other stimuli, for controlled *in situ* release of immunoadjuvant payload, directly into the tumor. The SRBs' release kinetics can be customized or programmed for sustained release compared to repeated systemic administration [28]. The use of SRBs could thus be optimized to significantly enhance local and metastatic tumor cell kill during RT with minimal toxicity or side effects for patients. Such an innovative approach could transform RT practice extending the use of RT to treatment of metastatic disease, hence many more patients.

Reducing treatment time or healthcare costs. With increasing advances in RT from conformal to IGRT and proton therapy, RT is considered by many as an expensive treatment modality, in particular in resource poor settings. Today, two-thirds of cancer deaths occur in LMICs. A drastic shortage of RT infrastructure in LMICs means that up to seventy per cent of cancer patients in LMICs who may benefit from radiation medicine do not receive this essential curative or pain relieving treatment. The International Atomic Energy Agency (IAEA) has been working to bring together RT equipment suppliers and RT users in developing countries to help make RT infrastructure more affordable and/or accessible to LMIC populations. Given the vast disparities in disease burden between developed countries and LMICs, researchers are also working to accelerate the production of new health technologies that may help to bridge this gap. The National Cancer Institute Center for Global Health and others are now also increasing funding mechanisms to promote the development of lower cost technologies that can make treatments including RT more affordable in LMICs. Affordability is inextricably linked to value, quality, efficiency, equity, and accessibility. To this end the use of SRBs, which could boost RT dose locally, is being considered as an approach to enable hypofractionation, which could in turn potentially reduce treatment times or healthcare costs. The use of SRBs to leverage the abscopal effect in treating metastatic disease is also an attractive approach that could benefit many more patients and increase survival, allowing for greater return on investment. This would yield major benefits in developing countries where patients often present with cancer already at the late stages. Partnerships or collaborations will be very important in this effort to develop lower cost technologies or adaptations of these that are more affordable. Pioneering efforts developing the use of SRBs in this direction are currently in progress [114].

Some researchers, such as Baumann *et al* [115] suggest that with recent technological advances in RT, new research and developments should focus less on improving the dose distribution and more on reducing treatment times [116]. If the use of SRBs for radiation boosting or priming the abscopal effect can lead to hypofractionation, the anticipated benefit of reducing healthcare costs is thus arguably justifiable. This is supported by recent studies [117] showing that use of hypofractionation results in a significant reduction in the financial costs associated with treating breast cancer patients.

In perspective, such an application aims to provide the equivalent effect of SABR. Here, instead of treating patients with many fractions, these low cost devices could literally replace currently used RT biomaterials (e.g. fiducials and spacers) for highly localized radiation boosting with minimal toxicity to healthy tissues [26]. From this perspective, this could again greatly benefit patients in LMICs because the wait times can be so long for many patients, even after trekking hundreds of miles to an RT center. The dearth or lack of RT units in many LMICs causes prolonged waiting times for receiving treatment and can even affect the timing between the administration of RT doses, hence compromising clinical outcomes and treatment effectiveness. In carrying out research for SRB technology applications in lower-cost RT, collaborations with developing country partners could be highly beneficial.

3.3.2.3 Future prospects

While one cannot predict the future, there are a number of logical directions where one could see further research and development beyond those highlighted above. Combining RT with other treatment modalities is a promising technique for increasing the cancer therapeutics ratio [118–121]. One logical direction is intensified efforts in the use of SBMs loaded with chemotherapy drugs. This could benefit patients eligible for concomitant chemoradiotherapy with minimal toxicities as described above. SRBs loading chemotherapy drugs with a high atomic number platinum component that can enhance RT, but also enable delivery of chemotherapy with minimal systemic toxicity, is an attractive area of research. Nanoparticles of such high atomic number for anticancer drugs have already been developed, including those of cisplatin, carboplatin, and oxaliplatain administered as adjuvants to brachytherapy or external beam RT [52–54, 122–124].

The prospect of increased collaborations to extend RT to systemic therapy via the abscopal effect is exciting and attractive and SRBs provide an opportunity for further R&D in combining RT and immunotherapy via an approach with such a rationale [119, 125–129]. SRBs eluting immunotherapy agents may provide a means of achieving greater effectiveness, and overcoming systematic toxicity due to intravenous administration, and also increasing accumulation of these agents at the tumor site or draining lymph nodes, since the agents are delivered locally within the tumor region [130]. Optimizing outcomes in combining RT with immunotherapy agents as a treatment modality may depend on the clear understanding of the nature of the tumor microenvironment, the effect of the agents on the tumor, as well as the radiation on the tumor after the application of the agent. For instance, how oxygenation or reactive oxygen species or immune cell populations vary within the tumor over the period of exposure to the agents and RT dosing [129, 131]. The mechanisms of radiation interacting with immunotherapy agents may be complex, as well as the interaction between the tumor and the targeting agents. Greater understanding of these complexities, including dosing, fractionation, and immunoadjuvants among other factors, is a growing area of research [129, 131, 132].

Cancer immunity consists of a number of key steps [76, 110], including release of antigens from tumor beds (which can be achieved with RT), presentation of tumor antigens by antigen-presenting cells (APCs), priming and activation of T-cells by activated APCs, migration and infiltration of effector T-cells back to the tumor, and finally the recognition and killing of tumor cells by effector T-cells. Each of these steps are targets with various therapeutic approaches. SRBs could employ different payloads targeting any of these steps. The ability of cancer cells to respond to the biomaterial in a controllable manner will be important in successful cancer treatments using SRBs. Signaling molecules are important and so cytokines could also be included in SRBs, e.g. Interferon gamma (IFNγ). IFNγ promotes macrophage repolarization and NK cell activation, and has been extensively studied as a promising adjuvant in vaccines, but its rapid clearance and systemic toxicity has severely limited its clinical efficacy [133]. The sustained *in situ* delivery via SRBs could overcome this limitation. There is probably going to be a growth in the number of studies using different immunoadjuvants targeting the different steps.

Another potential direction of R&D in SRBs is in the concomitant labeling of cancer cells. SRBs could be used to label cancer cells *in situ*, right at the source tumor. This may have significant advantages. An example motivating research in this direction is cancer metastasis, which accounts for over 90% of cancer associated suffering and death [134], involving circulating tumor cells (CTCs) shed by the primary tumor into the blood vessels or lymph nodes. The detection of such CTCs is valued in cancer management to monitor disease progression, tumor aggressiveness or treatment response. However, current methods to detect CTCs are limited by the scarcity of the CTCs in blood [135]. Only 1–10 CTCs are present in 1 ml of blood, which contains millions of white blood cells and almost a billion red blood cells [136]. As such, the direct detection of metastatic or rare CTCs remains a formidable technological problem when using currently available methods. For example, although the detection of the CTCs in lymph nodes is an attractive approach in diagnosing how aggressive a tumor is, the methods to do so are mostly suboptimal, accompanied by significant morbidities [136]. For instance, computed tomography and magnetic resonance imaging (MRI) are common and useful methods to detect anatomical abnormalities; however, they do not have the ability to differentiate between adenopathy related to inflammation and that caused by deposition of CTCs [137]. Currently other methods, e.g. cell counting, photoacoustic or fluorescence methods, Raman spectroscopy, and flow cytometry, which depend on CTC enrichment, are being developed [138–140]. Other approaches include the use of nanomaterials such as magnetic nanoparticles and carbon nanotubes for detecting and capturing CTCs [141–146].

The approach to label tumor cells *in situ* using SRBs may have a significant advantage over competing or current approaches. Since implantation of inert RT biomaterials is already part of current RT practice, replacing the inert biomaterials with the SRBs, loaded with NPs for sustained *in situ* release, will come at virtually no additional inconvenience to patients. Any labeled cell that may escape into the blood stream or lymph nodes may be tracked via a number of imaging methods, e.g. MRI or photoacoustic imaging. The ability to label CTCs *in situ* has the potential to significantly enhance the tracking, detection, and isolation efficiency of CTCs, and non-invasive nodal status assessment for cancer patients. Considering the fact that the nanoparticles are relatively non-toxic [40–42], this approach represents a potential low-risk high-reward approach compared to other approaches, which try to administer nanoparticles intravenously or find and label CTCs after they are already in circulation [147]. In addition, the ability to track CTCs right from the source, via either blood vessel or lymph node routes, as far as to distant metastatic sites could enhance overall understanding of cancer progression or metastasis. The approach could also complement nanoparticle-aided RT [26, 148] as more research considers cellular uptake of nanoparticles and their behavior as labels for localization microscopy that could benefit research and development in this area. GNPs could be suitable for imaging with nanometer resolution, and systematic counting of GNPs becomes feasible, because optical absorption and plasmon resonance effects result in optical blinking of GNPs at a size-dependent wavelength. SRBs loaded with gadolinium nanoparticles (e.g., Gd_2O_3, GdF_3, etc), when released, can also act as an MRI contrast agent, and a therapeutic agent for radiosensitization [60, 150–155]. Gadolinium-based nanoparticles are currently used as multimodal imaging agents for scintigraphy, computed tomography, and fluorescence imaging studies [156–159]. Radiolabeled nanoparticles (e.g. radiolabeled iron oxide), can also be incorporated into SRBs since they are promising agents for diagnostic applications [160].

Lower cost technologies have the potential to change the lives of millions of individuals living in LMICs and other resource-poor settings. With the emerging global radiation oncology movement, physicists, biologists, mathematicians, chemists, engineers, physicians, and other scientists will probably also now focus on developing lower cost technologies or adaptations of current technologies that can make RT more affordable and accessible in such settings. In the effort to develop lower cost technology, collaborations with LMIC partners will be strongly encouraged as done by the USA National Cancer Institute, with appropriate feedback to optimize the application. The development of these technologies should be based on co-creation with specific end-user adoptability and feedback. These should be incorporated to optimize designs so that effectiveness and durability in the intended clinical setting is ensured. Collaborations and co-creation with LMIC end-users can be powerful in allowing collaborators from various disciplines, institutions, and sectors to innovate around the challenges currently faced in global radiation oncology.

There are indubitably other potential applications that will emerge from the development of SRBs. Those highlighted in these review may not be comprehensive but provide a useful reference, in particular for cross-disciplinary collaborations towards the development and translation of such technologies. Creating opportunities and training programs for cross-disciplinary research for individuals engaged in these areas should also be encouraged to significantly accelerate the advancement of SRBs, facilitate clinical translation, and create new applications.

3.3.2.4 Conclusion

Biomaterials have already had an enormous impact on healthcare, as seen in myriad prosthetic and drug delivery device applications. Research on SRBs is still in its early days, but there is a strong rationale for upgrading the currently used inert RT biomaterials to smarter ones or developing stimuli-responsive nanoparticles that can deliver additional therapy enhancement benefits during RT. The anticipated range of applications for such smart devices could lead to increased survival and quality of life for cancer patients, and extend the benefits of RT to many more patients including in many LMICs. Current work is laying the foundations for significant advances in the development and potential clinical translation of SRBs. Cross-disciplinary and international collaborations could highly avail the development of the different applications in this area.

References

[1] NEPAD (New Partnership for Africa's Development, office of Science and Technology) 2006 *Africa's Science and Technology Consolidated Plan of Action* (Pretoria: NEPAD)

[2] Global status report on noncommunicable diseases 2010 www.who.int/nmh/publications/ncd_report_full_en.pdf Accessed June 20, 2017

[3] World Bank Country and Lending Groups World Bank Data Help Desk https://datahelpdesk.worldbank.org/knowledgebase/articles/906519-world-bank-country-and-lending-groups

[4] ASCO/AACR Methods in Clinical Cancer Research Workshop www.aacr.org/Meetings/Pages/MeetingDetail.aspx?EventItemID=111&utm_source=social&utm_medium=facebook&utm_campaign=workshop#.WUp9v4zyuUk Accessed June 21, 2017

[5] Cancer Institute N. CANCER: Changing the Conversation, The Nation's Investment in Cancer Research, An Annual Plan and Budget Proposal for Fiscal Year 2012 www.cancer.gov/about-nci/budget/annual-plan/nci-plan-2012.pdf Accessed June 20, 2017

[6] Ngwa W *et al* 2017 Potential role of the quality assurance review center (QARC) platform in Global Radiation Oncology *Int. J. Radiat. Oncol. Biol. Phys.* https://doi.org/ROB24395 in press

[7] Ngwa W *et al* 2016 Closing the cancer divide through ubuntu: information and communication technology-powered models for global radiation oncology *Int. J. Radiat. Oncol. Biol. Phys.* **94** 440–9

[8] Ngwa W *et al* 2015 Potential for information and communication technologies to catalyze global collaborations in radiation oncology *Int. J. Radiat. Oncol. Biol. Phys.* **91** 444–7

[9] Ngwa W and Ngoma T 2016 *Emerging Models for Global Health in Radiation Oncology* (Bristol: IOP Publishing)

[10] FitzGerald T J 2014 A new model for imaging and radiation therapy quality assurance in the National Clinical Trials Network of the National Cancer Institute *Int. J. Radiat. Oncol. Biol. Phys.* **88** 272–3

[11] Fitzgerald T J *et al* 2013 Future vision for the quality assurance of oncology clinical trials *Front. Oncol.* **3** 31

[12] Deasy J O, Blanco A I and Clark V H 2003 CERR: a computational environment for radiotherapy research *Med. Phys.* **30** 979–85

[13] Coelho K R 2012 Challenges of the oral cancer burden in India *J. Cancer Epidemiol.* **2012** 701932

[14] Hempstead J *et al* 2015 Low-cost photodynamic therapy devices for global health settings: characterization of battery-powered LED performance and smartphone imaging in 3D tumor models *Sci. Rep.* **5**

[15] Mallidi S *et al* 2015 *In vivo* evaluation of battery-operated light-emitting diode-based photodynamic therapy efficacy using tumor volume and biomarker expression as endpoints *J. Biomed. Opt.* **20** 048003

[16] Atun R *et al* 2015 Expanding global access to radiotherapy *Lancet Oncol.* **16** 1153–86

[17] Canter D, Greenberg R E, Horwitz E M, Kutikov A, Li J, Long C, Buyyounouski M and Boorjian S A 2010 Implantation of electromagnetic transponders following radical prostatectomy for delivery of *IMRT. Can. J. Urol.* **17** 5365–9

[18] Balter J M, Wright J N, Newell L J, Friemel B, Dimmer S, Cheng Y, Wong J, Vertatschitsch E and Mate T P 2005 Accuracy of a wireless localization system for radiotherapy *Int. J. Radiat. Oncol. Biol. Phys.* **61** 933–7

[19] Ng M, Brown E, Williams A, Chao M, Lawrentschuk N and Chee R 2014 Fiducial markers and spacers in prostate radiotherapy: current applications *BJU Int.* **113** Suppl 2 13–20

[20] Shirato H *et al* 2003 Feasibility of insertion/implantation of 2.0-mm-diameter gold internal fiducial markers for precise setup and real-time tumor tracking in radiotherapy *Int. J. Radiat. Oncol. Biol. Phys.* **56** 240–7

[21] van der Heide U A, Kotte A N, Dehnad H, Hofman P, Lagenijk J J and van Vulpen M 2007 Analysis of fiducial marker-based position verification in the external beam radiotherapy of patients with prostate cancer *Radiother. Oncol.* **82** 38–45

[22] Khashab M A *et al* 2012 Comparative analysis of traditional and coiled fiducials implanted during EUS for pancreatic cancer patients receiving stereotactic body radiation therapy *Gastrointest. Endosc.* **76** 962–71

[23] Dempsey J F, Williams J A, Stubbs J B, Patrick T J and Williamson J F 1998 Dosimetric properties of a novel brachytherapy balloon applicator for the treatment of malignant brain-tumor resection-cavity margins *Int. J. Radiat. Oncol. Biol. Phys.* **42** 421–9

[24] Segala J J, Cardarelli G A, Hiatt J R, Curran B H and Sternick E S 2011 Interface dosimetry for electronic brachytherapy intracavitary breast balloon applicators *J. Appl. Clin. Med. Phys.* **12** 3221

[25] Choi J H, Seo D W, Park do H, Lee S K and Kim M H 2014 Fiducial placement for stereotactic body radiation therapy under only endoscopic ultrasonography guidance in pancreatic and hepatic malignancy: practical feasibility and safety *Gut Liver* **8** 88–93

[26] Ngwa W, Kumar R, Sridhar S, Korideck H, Zygmanski P, Cormack R A, Berbeco R and Makrigiorgos G M 2014 Targeted radiotherapy with gold nanoparticles: current status and future perspectives *Nanomedicine* **9** 1063–82

[27] Kumar R, Belz J, Markovic S, Jadhav T, Fowle W, Niedre M, Cormack R, Makrigiorgos M G and Sridhar S 2015 Nanoparticle-based brachytherapy spacers for delivery of localized combined chemoradiation therapy *Int. J. Radiat. Oncol. Biol. Phys.* **91** 393–400

[28] Nagesha D K, Tada D B, Stambaugh C K, Gultepe E, Jost E, Levy C O, Cormack R, Makrigiorgos G M and Sridhar S 2010 Radiosensitizer-eluting nanocoatings on gold fiducials for biological *in situ* image-guided radio therapy (BIS-IGRT) *Phys. Med. Biol.* **55** 6039–52

[29] Sinha N, Cifter G, Sajo E, Kumar R, Sridhar S, Nguyen P L, Cormack R A, Makrigiorgos G M and Ngwa W 2015 Brachytherapy application with *in situ* dose painting administered by gold nanoparticle eluters *Int. J. Radiat. Oncol. Biol. Phys.* **91** 385–92

[30] Cormack R A, Sridhar S, Suh W W, D'Amico A V and Makrigiorgos G M 2010 Biological *in situ* dose painting for image-guided radiation therapy using drug-loaded implantable devices *Int. J. Radiat. Oncol. Biol. Phys.* **76** 615–23

[31] Shinohara K and Roach M 2008 Technique for implantation of fiducial markers in the prostate *Urology* **71** 196–200

[32] Langer R and Tirrell D A 2004 Designing materials for biology and medicine *Nature* **428** 487-92

[33] Ulery B D, Nair L S and Laurencin C T 2011 Biomedical applications of biodegradable polymers *J. Polym. Sci.* B **49** 832–64

[34] Anderson D G, Burdick J A and Langer R 2004 Materials science. Smart biomaterials *Science* **305** 1923–4

[35] Mieszawska A J and Kaplan D L 2010 Smart biomaterials—regulating cell behavior through signaling molecules *BMC Biol.* **8** 59

[36] Perez R A, Won J E, Knowles J C and Kim H W 2013 Naturally and synthetic smart composite biomaterials for tissue regeneration *Adv. Drug Deliv. Rev.* **65** 471–96

[37] Cifter G, Chin J, Cifter F, Altundal Y, Sinha N, Sajo E and Ngwa W 2015 Targeted radiotherapy enhancement during electronic brachytherapy of accelerated partial breast irradiation (APBI) using controlled release of gold nanoparticles *Phys. Medica* **31** 1070–4

[38] Ouyang Z, Mainali M K, Sinha N, Strack G, Altundal Y, Hao Y, Winningham T A, Sajo E, Celli J and Ngwa W 2016 Potential of using cerium oxide nanoparticles for protecting healthy tissue during accelerated partial breast irradiation (APBI) *Phys. Medica* **32** 631–5

[39] Freeman T 2015 Smart implants tackle metastatic disease *Med. Phys. Web* September 9 http://medicalphysicsweb.org/cws/article/research/62482

[40] Lasagna-Reeves C, Gonzalez-Romero D, Barria M A, Olmedo I, Clos A, Sadagopa Ramanujam V M, Urayama A, Vergara L, Kogan M J and Soto C 2010 Bioaccumulation and toxicity of gold nanoparticles after repeated administration in mice *Biochem. Biophys. Res. Commun.* **393** 649–55

[41] Mukherjee P, Bhattacharya R, Wang P, Wang L, Basu S, Nagy J A, Atala A, Mukhopadhyay D and Soker S 2005 Antiangiogenic properties of gold nanoparticles *Clin. Cancer Res.* **11** 3530–4

[42] Shukla R, Bansal V, Chaudhary M, Basu A, Bhonde R R and Sastry M 2005 Biocompatibility of gold nanoparticles and their endocytotic fate inside the cellular compartment: a microscopic overview *Langmuir* **21** 10644–54

[43] Fransen M F, Cordfunke R A, Sluijter M, van Steenbergen M J, Drijfhout J W, Ossendorp F, Hennink W E and Melief C J 2014 Effectiveness of slow-release systems in CD40 agonistic antibody immunotherapy of cancer *Vaccine* **32** 1654–60

[44] Sandin L C, Orlova A, Gustafsson E, Ellmark P, Tolmachev V, Totterman T H and Mangsbo S M 2014 Locally delivered CD40 agonist antibody accumulates in secondary lymphoid organs and eradicates experimental disseminated bladder cancer *Cancer Immunol. Res.* **2** 80–90

[45] Sandin L C, Totterman T H and Mangsbo S M 2014 Local immunotherapy based on agonistic CD40 antibodies effectively inhibits experimental bladder cancer *Oncoimmunology* **3** e27400

[46] Kumar R, Korideck H, Ngwa W, Berbeco R I, Makrigiorgos G M and Sridhar S 2103 Third generation gold nanoplatform optimized for radiation therapy *Transl. Cancer Res.* **2**

[47] Burger N, Biswas A, Barzan D, Kirchner A, Hosser H, Hausmann M, Hildenbrand G, Herskind C, Wenz F and Veldwijk M R 2014 A method for the efficient cellular uptake and retention of small modified gold nanoparticles for the radiosensitization of cells *Nanomedicine* **10** 1365–73

[48] Sullivan L B and Chandel N S 2014 Mitochondrial reactive oxygen species and cancer *Cancer Metab.* **2** 17

[49] Cao W, Cudney H H and Waser R 1999 Smart materials and structures *Proc. Natl Acad. Sci. USA* **96** 8330–1

[50] Tada D B, Singh S, Nagesha D, Jost E, Levy C O, Gultepe E, Cormack R, Makrigiorgos G M and Sridhar S 2010 Chitosan film containing poly(D,L-lactic-co-glycolic acid) nanoparticles: a platform for localized dual-drug release *Pharm. Res.* **27** 1738–45

[51] Markovic S, Belz J, Kumar R, Cormack R A, Sridhar S and Niedre M 2016 Near-infrared fluorescence imaging platform for quantifying *in vivo* nanoparticle diffusion from drug loaded implants *Int. J. Nanomed.* **11** 1213–23

[52] Altundal Y, Cifter G, Detappe A, Sajo E, Tsiamas P, Zygmanski P, Berbeco R, Cormack R A, Makrigiorgos M and Ngwa W 2015 New potential for enhancing concomitant chemoradiotherapy with FDA approved concentrations of cisplatin via the photoelectric effect *Phys. Medica* **31** 25–30

[53] Hao Y, Altundal Y, Moreau M, Sajo E, Kumar R and Ngwa W 2015 Potential for enhancing external beam radiotherapy for lung cancer using high-Z nanoparticles administered via inhalation *Phys. Med. Biol.* **60** 7035–43

[54] Cifter G, Altundal Y, Detappe A, Sajo E, Berbeco R, Makrigiorgos M and Ngwa W 2015 Dose enhancement during concomitant chemoradiotherapy using FDA approved concentrations of carboplatin and oxaliplatin nanoparticles *World Congr. on Medical Physics and Biomedical Engineering (June 7–12, Toronto, Canada)* ed A D Jaffray (Cham: Springer) pp 1723–6

[55] Schuemann J, Berbeco R, Chithrani D B, Cho S H, Kumar R, McMahon S J, Sridhar S and Krishnan S 2016 Roadmap to clinical use of gold nanoparticles for radiation sensitization *Int. J. Radiat. Oncol. Biol. Phys.* **94** 189–205

[56] Rancoule C, Magne N, Vallard A, Guy J B, Rodriguez-Lafrasse C, Deutsch E and Chargari C 2015 Nanoparticles in radiation oncology: from bench-side to bedside *Cancer Lett.* **375** 256–62
[57] Baetke S C, Lammers T and Kiessling F 2015 Applications of nanoparticles for diagnosis and therapy of cancer *Br. J. Radiol.* **88** 20150207
[58] Jain S, Hirst D G and O'Sullivan J M 2012 Gold nanoparticles as novel agents for cancer therapy *Br. J. Radiol.* **85** 101–13
[59] Prise K M and Martin S G 2015 Editorial-nanoparticles for diagnostic imaging and radiotherapy *Br. J. Radiol.* **88** 20150692
[60] Lux F, Sancey L, Bianchi A, Cremillieux Y, Roux S and Tillement O 2015 Gadolinium-based nanoparticles for theranostic MRI-radiosensitization *Nanomedicine* **10** 1801–15
[61] Pottier A, Borghi E and Levy L 2015 The future of nanosized radiation enhancers *Br. J. Radiol.* **88** 20150171
[62] Friedman A D, Claypool S E and Liu R 2013 The smart targeting of nanoparticles *Curr. Pharm. Des.* **19** 6315–29
[63] Nicol J R, Dixon D and Coulter J A 2015 Gold nanoparticle surface functionalization: a necessary requirement in the development of novel nanotherapeutics *Nanomedicine* **10** 1315–26
[64] Boisselier E and Astruc D 2009 Gold nanoparticles in nanomedicine: preparations, imaging, diagnostics, therapies and toxicity *Chem. Soc. Rev.* **38** 1759–82
[65] Mieszawska A J, Mulder W J, Fayad Z A and Cormode D P 2013 Multifunctional gold nanoparticles for diagnosis and therapy of disease *Molec. Pharma.* **10** 831–47
[66] Curry T, Kopelman R, Shilo M and Popovtzer R 2014 Multifunctional theranostic gold nanoparticles for targeted CT imaging and photothermal therapy *Contrast Media Molec. Imag.* **9** 53–61
[67] de Barros A B, Tsourkas A, Saboury B, Cardoso V N and Alavi A 2012 Emerging role of radiolabeled nanoparticles as an effective diagnostic technique *EJNMMI Res.* **2** 39
[68] Kim B, Han G, Toley B J, Kim C K, Rotello V M and Forbes N S 2010 Tuning payload delivery in tumour cylindroids using gold nanoparticles *Nat. Nanotechnol.* **5** 465–72
[69] Allemann E, Brasseur N, Benrezzak O, Rousseau J, Kudrevich S V, Boyle R W, Leroux J C, Gurny R and Van Lier J E 1995 PEG-coated poly(lactic acid) nanoparticles for the delivery of hexadecafluoro zinc phthalocyanine to EMT-6 mouse mammary tumours *J. Pharmacy Pharmacol.* **47** 382–7
[70] Fredman G, Kamaly N, Spolitu S, Milton J, Ghorpade D, Chiasson R, Kuriakose G, Perretti M, Farokhzad O and Tabas I 2015 Targeted nanoparticles containing the proresolving peptide Ac2-26 protect against advanced atherosclerosis in hypercholesterolemic mice *Sci. Transl. Med.* **7** 275ra20
[71] Erathodiyil N and Ying J Y 2011 Functionalization of inorganic nanoparticles for bioimaging applications *Acc. Chem. Res.* **44** 925–35
[72] Maeda H, Sawa T and Konno T 2011 Mechanism of tumor-targeted delivery of macromolecular drugs, including the EPR effect in solid tumor and clinical overview of the prototype polymeric drug SMANCS *J. Control. Release* **74** 47–61
[73] Fang J, Sawa T and Maeda H 2003 Factors and mechanism of 'EPR' effect and the enhanced antitumor effects of macromolecular drugs including SMANCS *Adv. Exper. Med. Biol.* **519** 29–49

[74] Mura S, Nicolas J and Couvreur P 2013 Stimuli-responsive nanocarriers for drug delivery *Nat. Mater.* **12** 991–1003

[75] Fan Y and Moon J J 2015 Nanoparticle drug delivery systems designed to improve cancer vaccines and immunotherapy *Vaccines* 3:662–85

[76] Saluja S S, Hanlon D J, Sharp F A, Hong E, Khalil D, Robinson E, Tigelaar R and Fahmy T M; Edelson R L 2014 Targeting human dendritic cells via DEC-205 using PLGA nanoparticles leads to enhanced cross-presentation of a melanoma-associated antigen *Int. J. Nanomed.* **9** 5231–46

[77] Mitra A, Nan A, Line B R and Ghandehari H 2006 Nanocarriers for nuclear imaging and radiotherapy of cancer *Current Pharma. Des.* **12** 4729–49

[78] Ting G, Chang C H, Wang H E and Lee T W 2010 Nanotargeted radionuclides for cancer nuclear imaging and internal radiotherapy *J. Biomed. Biotechnol.* **2010** 953537

[79] Chang C H, Stabin M G, Chang Y J, Chen L C, Chen M H, Chang T J, Lee T W and Ting G 2008 Comparative dosimetric evaluation of nanotargeted (188)Re-(DXR)-liposome for internal radiotherapy *Cancer Biother. Radiopharmaceut.* **23** 749–58

[80] Lammers T, Kiessling F, Hennink W E and Storm G 2010 Nanotheranostics and image-guided drug delivery: current concepts and future directions *Molec. Pharmaceut.* **7** 1899–912

[81] Muthu M S, Leong D T, Mei L and Feng S S 2014 Nanotheranostics—application and further development of nanomedicine strategies for advanced theranostics *Theranostics* **4** 660–77

[82] Song J, Kim J, Hwang S, Jeon M, Jeong S, Kim C and Kim S 2016 'Smart' gold nanoparticles for photoacoustic imaging: an imaging contrast agent responsive to the cancer microenvironment and signal amplification via pH-induced aggregation *Chem. Commun. (Camb)* **52** 8287–90

[83] Wong C, Stylianopoulos T, Cui J, Martin J, Chauhan V P, Jiang W, Popovic Z, Jain R K, Bawendi M G and Fukumura D 2011 Multistage nanoparticle delivery system for deep penetration into tumor tissue *Proc. Natl Acad. Sci. USA* **108** 2426–31

[84] Zhang D G, Feygelman V, Moros E G, Latifi K and Zhang G G 2014 Monte Carlo study of radiation dose enhancement by gadolinium in megavoltage and high dose rate radiotherapy *PloSone* **9** e109389

[85] Kim T J, Chae K S, Chang Y and Lee G H 2013 Gadolinium oxide nanoparticles as potential multimodal imaging and therapeutic agents *Curr. Top. Med. Chem.* **13** 422–33

[86] Yang X L, Ju X J, Mu X T, Wang W, Xie R, Liu Z and Chu L Y 2016 core–shell chitosan microcapsules for programmed sequential drug release *ACS Appl. Mater. Interfaces* **8** 10524–34

[87] Yang Y S, Carney R P, Stellacci F and Irvine D J 2014 Enhancing radiotherapy by lipid nanocapsule-mediated delivery of amphiphilic gold nanoparticles to intracellular membranes *ACS Nano* **8** 8992–9002

[88] Park H K, Lee S J, Oh J S, Lee S G, Jeong Y I and Lee H C 2015 Smart nanoparticles based on hyaluronic acid for redox-responsive and CD44 receptor-mediated targeting of tumor *Nanoscale Res. Lett.* **10** 981

[89] Poojari R J 2013 PLGA: the smart therapeutics goods carrier *Front. Pharmacol.* **4** 20

[90] Priya James H, John R, Alex A and Anoop K R 2014 Smart polymers for the controlled delivery of drugs—a concise overview *Acta Pharm. Sin.* B **4** 120–7

[91] Egunov A I, Inaba A, Gree S, Malval J P, Tamura K, Saito Y and Luchnikov V A 2016 Time-programmed release of fluoroscein isocyanate dextran from micro-pattern-designed polymer scrolls *J. Control. Release* **233** 39–47
[92] Park J and Babensee J E 2012 Differential functional effects of biomaterials on dendritic cell maturation *Acta Biomater.* **8** 3606–17
[93] Lendlein A, Jiang H, Junger O and Langer R 2005 Light-induced shape-memory polymers *Nature* **434** 879–82
[94] Adhikary R R, More P and Banerjee R 2015 Smart nanoparticles as targeting platforms for HIV infections *Nanoscale* **7** 7520–34
[95] Lutz E R *et al* 2014 Immunotherapy converts nonimmunogenic pancreatic tumors into immunogenic foci of immune regulation *Cancer Immunol. Res.* **2** 616–31
[96] Ngwa W, Kumar R, Sridhar S, Korideck H, Zygmanski P, Cormack R C, Berbeco R I and Makrigiorgos G M 2016 Targeted radiotherapy with gold nanoparticles: current status and future perspectives *Nanomedicine* **9** 1063–82
[97] Purdy J A 2008 Dose to normal tissues outside the radiation therapy patient's treated volume: a review of different radiation therapy techniques *Health Phys.* **95** 666–76
[98] Button M R and Staffurth J N 2010 Clinical application of image-guided radiotherapy in bladder and prostate cancer *Clin. Oncol.* **22** 698–706
[99] Milas L, Murray D, Brock W A and Meyn R E 1988 Radioprotectors in tumor radiotherapy: factors and settings determining therapeutic ratio *Pharma. Ther.* **39** 179–87
[100] Keall P J *et al* 2006 The management of respiratory motion in radiation oncology: report of AAPM Task Group 76 *Med. Phys.* **33** 3874–900
[101] Machtay M, Bae K, Movsas B, Paulus R, Gore E M, Komaki R, Albain K, Sause W T and Curran W J 2012 Higher biologically effective dose of radiotherapy is associated with improved outcomes for locally advanced non-small cell lung carcinoma treated with chemoradiation: an analysis of the Radiation Therapy Oncology Group *Int. J. Radiat. Oncol. Biol. Phys.* **82** 425–34
[102] Hainfeld J F, Slatkin D N and Smilowitz H M 2004 The use of gold nanoparticles to enhance radiotherapy in mice *Phys. Med. Biol.* **49** N309–15
[103] Berbeco R I, Korideck H, Ngwa W, Kumar R, Patel J, Sridhar S, Johnson S, Price B D, Kimmelman A and Makrigiorgos G M 2012 DNA damage enhancement from gold nanoparticles for clinical MV photon beams *Radiat. Res.* **178** 604–8
[104] Ngwa W, Korideck H, Kassis A I, Kumar R, Sridhar S, Makrigiorgos G M and Cormack R A 2013 *In vitro* radiosensitization by gold nanoparticles during continuous low-dose-rate gamma irradiation with I-125 brachytherapy seeds *Nanomedicine* **9** 25–7
[105] Perrault S D and Chan W C 2010 *In vivo* assembly of nanoparticle components to improve targeted cancer imaging *Proc. Natl Acad. Sci. USA* **107** 11194–9
[106] Mole R H 1953 Whole body irradiation; radiobiology or medicine? *Br. J. Radiol.* **26** 234–41
[107] Demaria S, Ng B, Devitt M L, Babb J S, Kawashima N, Liebes L and Formenti S C 2004 Ionizing radiation inhibition of distant untreated tumors (abscopal effect) is immune *mediated Int. J. Radiat. Oncol. Biol. Phys.* **58** 862–70
[108] Tang C *et al* 2014 Combining radiation and immunotherapy: a new systemic therapy for solid tumors? *Cancer Immunol. Res.* **2** 831–8
[109] Formenti S C and Demaria S 2009 Systemic effects of local radiotherapy *Lancet Oncol.* **10** 718–26

[110] Golden E B *et al* 2015 Local radiotherapy and granulocyte-macrophage colony-stimulating factor to generate abscopal responses in patients with metastatic solid tumours: a proof-of-principle trial *Lancet Oncol.* **16** 795–803
[111] Vanpouille-Box C, Pilones K A, Wennerberg E, Formenti S C and Demaria S 2015 *In situ* vaccination by radiotherapy to improve responses to anti-CTLA-4 treatment *Vaccine* **33** 7415–22
[112] Marabelle A, Kohrt H, Caux C and Levy R 2014 Intratumoral immunization: a new paradigm for cancer therapy *Clin. Cancer Res.* **20** 1747–56
[113] Golden E B, Demaria S, Schiff P B, Chachoua A and Formenti S C 2013 An abscopal response to radiation and ipilimumab in a patient with metastatic non-small cell lung cancer *Cancer Immunol. Res.* **1** 365–72
[114] TiDTiC www.tidtac.org: TiDTaC Accessed January 2016
[115] Baumann M, Krause M, Overgaard J, Debus J, Bentzen S M, Daartz J, Richter C, Zips D and Bortfeld T 2016 Radiation oncology in the era of precision medicine *Nat. Rev. Cancer* **16** 234–49
[116] Arcangeli S and Greco C 2016 Hypofractionated radiotherapy for organ-confined prostate cancer: is less more? *Nat. Rev. Urol.* **13** 400–8
[117] Mortimer J W, McLachlan C S, Hansen C J, Assareh H, Last A, McKay M J and Shakespeare T P 2016 Use of hypofractionated post-mastectomy radiotherapy reduces health costs by over $2000 per patient: an Australian perspective *J. Med. Imaging Radiat. Oncol.* **60** 146–53
[118] LaRue S M and Vujaskovic Z 1995 Combining radiation therapy with other treatment modalities *Seminars Vet. Med. Surg.* **10** 197–204
[119] Hodge J W, Guha C, Neefjes J and Gulley J L 2008 Synergizing radiation therapy and immunotherapy for curing incurable cancers. Opportunities and challenges *Oncology* **22** 1064–70 1075, 1080, 1081, 1084
[120] Page R L and Thrall D E 1990 Clinical indications and applications of radiotherapy and hyperthermia in veterinary oncology *Vet. Clin. North Am. Small Animal Pract.* **20** 1075–92
[121] Bernier J *et al* 2004 Postoperative irradiation with or without concomitant chemotherapy for locally advanced head and neck cancer *New England J. Med.* **350** 1945–52
[122] Peng X H *et al* 2011 Targeted delivery of cisplatin to lung cancer using ScFvEGFR-heparin-cisplatin nanoparticles *ACS Nano* **5** 9480–93
[123] Rousseau J, Barth R F, Fernandez M, Adam J F, Balosso J, Esteve F and Elleaume H 2010 Efficacy of intracerebral delivery of cisplatin in combination with photon irradiation for treatment of brain tumors *J. Neurooncol.* **98** 287–95
[124] Demaria S, Bhardwaj N, McBride W H and Formenti S C 2005 Combining radiotherapy and immunotherapy: a revived partnership *Int. J. Radiat. Oncol. Biol. Phys.* **63** 655–66
[125] Sharp H J, Wansley E K, Garnett C T, Chakraborty M, Camphausen K, Schlom J and Hodge J W 2007 Synergistic antitumor activity of immune strategies combined with radiation *Front. Biosci.* **12** 4900–10
[126] Kamrava M, Bernstein M B, Camphausen K and Hodge J W 2009 Combining radiation, immunotherapy, and antiangiogenesis agents in the management of cancer: the Three Musketeers or just another quixotic combination? *Molecular bioSystems* **5** 1262–70
[127] O'Reilly M S 2006 Radiation combined with antiangiogenic and antivascular agents *Semin. Radiat. Oncol.* **16** 45–50

[128] Wachsberger P, Burd R and Dicker A P 2003 Tumor response to ionizing radiation combined with antiangiogenesis or vascular targeting agents: exploring mechanisms of interaction *Clin. Cancer Res.* **9** 1957–71

[129] Hao Y, Cifter G, Altundal Y, Sinha N, Moreau M, Sajo E, Makrigiorgos G and Ngwa W 2015 MO-FG-BRA-04: leveraging the abscopal effect via new design radiotherapy biomaterials loaded with immune checkpoint inhibitors *Med. Phys.* **42** 3565

[130] Timke C, Zieher H, Roth A, Hauser K, Lipson K E, Weber K J, Debus J, Abdollahi A and Huber P E 2008 Combination of vascular endothelial growth factor receptor/platelet-derived growth factor receptor inhibition markedly improves radiation tumor therapy *Clin. Cancer Res.* **14** 2210–9

[131] Abdollahi A *et al* 2003 Combined therapy with direct and indirect angiogenesis inhibition results in enhanced antiangiogenic and antitumor effects *Cancer Res.* **63** 8890–8

[132] Segura S, Espuelas S, Renedo M J and Irache J M 2005 Potential of albumin nanoparticles as carriers for interferon gamma *Drug Dev. Ind. Pharm.* **31** 271–80

[133] Weigelt B, Peterse J L and Van't Veer L J 2005 Breast cancer metastasis: markers and models *Nature Rev. Cancer* **5** 591–602

[134] Wang X, Qian X, Beitler J J, Chen Z G, Khuri F R, Lewis M M, Shin H J C, Nie S and Shin D M 2011 Detection of circulating tumor cells in human peripheral blood using surface-enhanced Raman scattering nanoparticles *Cancer Res.* **71** 1526–32

[135] Miller M C, Doyle G V and Terstappen L W 2010 Significance of circulating tumor cells detected by the cellsearch system in patients with metastatic breast colorectal and prostate cancer *J. Oncol.* 2010 617421

[136] Nakagawa T, Martinez S R, Goto Y, Koyanagi K, Kitago M, Shingai T, Elashoff D A, Ye X, Singer F R and Giuliano A E 2007 Detection of circulating tumor cells in early-stage breast cancer metastasis to axillary lymph nodes *Clin. Cancer Res.* **13** 4105–10

[137] Fass L 2008 Imaging and cancer: a review *Molecular Oncol.* **2** 115–52

[138] Weight R M and Viator J A 2014 Detection of circulating tumor cells by photoacoustic flowmetry *Methods Mol. Biol.* **1102** 655–63

[139] Neugebauer U, Bocklitz T, Clement J H, Krafft C and Popp J 2010 Towards detection and identification of circulating tumour cells using Raman spectroscopy *Analyst* **135** 3178–82

[140] Georgakoudi I, Solban N, Novak J, Rice W L, Wei X, Hasan T and Lin C P 2004 *In vivo* flow cytometry: a new method for enumerating circulating cancer cells *Cancer Res.* **64** 5044–7

[141] Benez A, Geiselhart A, Handgretinger R, Schiebel U and Fierlbeck G 1999 Detection of circulating melanoma cells by immunomagnetic cell sorting *J. Clin. Lab. Anal.* **13** 229–33

[142] Georgakoudi I, Solban N, Novak J, Rice W L, Wei X, Hasan T and Lin C P 2004 *In vivo* flow cytometry a new method for enumerating circulating cancer cells *Cancer Res.* **64** 5044–7

[143] Hsieh H B, Marrinucci D, Bethel K, Curry D N, Humphrey M, Krivacic R T, Kroener J, Kroener L, Ladanyi A and Lazarus N 2006 High speed detection of circulating tumor cells *Biosensors Bioelectr.* **21** 1893–9

[144] Weight R M, Viator J A, Dale P S, Caldwell C W and Lisle A E 2006 Photoacoustic detection of metastatic melanoma cells in the human circulatory system *Opt. Lett.* **31** 2998–3000

[145] Chithrani B D, Ghazani A A and Chan W C 2006 Determining the size and shape dependence of gold nanoparticle uptake into mammalian cells *Nano Lett.* **6** 662–8

[146] Sha M Y, Xu H, Natan M J and Cromer R 2008 Surface-enhanced Raman scattering tags for rapid and homogeneous detection of circulating tumor cells in the presence of human whole blood *J. Am. Chem. Soc.* **130** 17214–5

[147] Galanzha E I, Shashkov E V, Kelly T, Kim J W, Yang L and Zharov V P 2009 *In vivo* magnetic enrichment and multiplex photoacoustic detection of circulating tumour cells *Nat. Nanotechnol.* **4** 855–60
[148] Moser F *et al* 2016 Cellular uptake of gold nanoparticles and their behavior as labels for localization microscopy *Biophys. J.* **110** 947–53
[149] Thomas R, Park I K and Jeong Y Y 2013 Magnetic iron oxide nanoparticles for multimodal imaging and therapy of cancer *Int. J. Mol. Sci.* **14** 15910–30
[150] Bouziotis P, Psimadas D, Tsotakos T, Stamopoulos D and Tsoukalas C 2012 Radiolabeled iron oxide nanoparticles as dual-modality SPECT/MRI and PET/MRI agents *Curr. Top. Med. Chem.* **12** 2694–702
[151] Le Duc G *et al* 2011 Toward an image-guided microbeam radiation therapy using gadolinium-based nanoparticles *ACS Nano* **5** 9566–74
[152] Le Duc G *et al* 2011 Toward an image-guided microbeam radiation therapy using gadolinium-based nanoparticles *ACS Nano* **5** 9566–74
[153] Faure A C, Dufort S, Josserand V, Perriat P, Coll J L, Roux S and Tillement O 2009 Control of the *in vivo* biodistribution of hybrid nanoparticles with different poly(ethylene glycol) coatings *Small* **5** 2565–75
[154] Bridot J L *et al* 2007 Hybrid gadolinium oxide nanoparticles: multimodal contrast agents for *in vivo* imaging *J. Am. Chem. Soc.* **129** 5076–84
[155] Ahmad M W, Xu W, Kim S J, Baeck J S, Chang Y, Bae J E, Chae K S, Park J A, Kim T J and Lee G H 2015 Potential dual imaging nanoparticle: Gd_2O_3 nanoparticle *Sci. Rep.* **5** 8549
[156] Kumar S, Meena V K, Hazari P P and Sharma R K 2016 FITC-Dextran entrapped and silica coated gadolinium oxide nanoparticles for synchronous optical and magnetic resonance imaging applications *Int. J. Pharma.* **506** 242–52
[157] Ghaghada K B, Ravoori M, Sabapathy D, Bankson J, Kundra V and Annapragada A 2009 New dual mode gadolinium nanoparticle contrast agent for magnetic resonance imaging *PLoS One* **4** e7628
[158] Misri R, Meier D, Yung A C, Kozlowski P and Hafeli U O 2012 Development and evaluation of a dual-modality (MRI/SPECT) molecular imaging bioprobe *Nanomedicine* **8** 1007–16
[159] Srivatsan A and Chen X 2014 Recent advances in nanoparticle-based nuclear imaging of cancers *Adv. Cancer Res.* **124** 83–129
[160] Xing Y, Zhao J, Conti P S and Chen K 2014 Radiolabeled nanoparticles for multimodality tumor imaging *Theranostics* **4** 290–306

Chapter 4

Global oncology care: until every cancer patient has access to treatment

Dow Wilson, Krish Suthanthiran, Franklin Huang, Samba Richard, Christian Ntizimira, Ahmed Elzawawy and Esther Ikiara

4.1 Expanding global access to radiotherapy

Lecture by Dow Wilson (President and CEO Varian Medical Systems)

4.1.1 Introduction

There is a growing burden of cancer in low and middle income countries (LMICs), and a changing burden of disease, e.g. in Africa (figure 4.1).

According to the World Health Organization (WHO), African cancer deaths are expected to increase from 320 000 to 967 000 per year with cancer greater than 25% of the predicted increase for all causes of death. The Lancet Oncology Commission released a report on expanding global access to radiotherapy, which is considered to be a cost effective treatment modality for cancer [1]. Over 50% of cancer patients need radiotherapy, but less than 10% of patients have access to radiotherapy in low

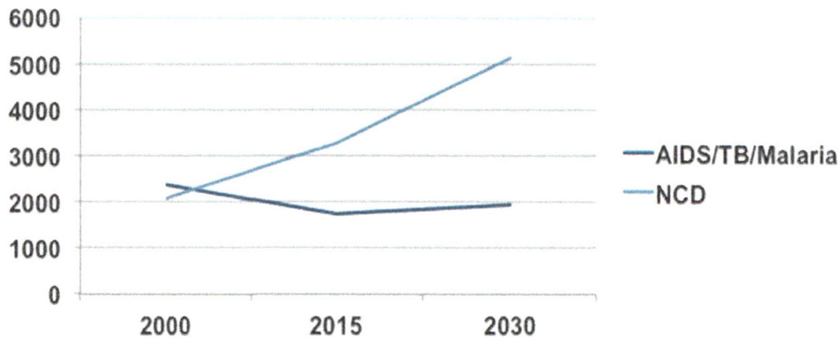

Figure 4.1. Mortality in thousands in Africa. NCD = non-communicable disease.

doi:10.1088/978-0-7503-1359-9ch4

income countries. According to the Lancet report, 26.9 million life years could be saved from scale-up of radiotherapy in LMICs from 2015 to 2035.

4.1.2 Lancet Commission call to action

To address the situation the Lancet Oncology Commission outlined the calls to action highlighted in table 4.1 [1].

Action 1 calls for population-based cancer control plans. These plans need to include radiotherapy as a crucial component of care. A goal is that by 2020, 80% of countries should have cancer control plans that include radiotherapy. A good example is Algeria, with a cancer control plan that aims to establish 13 new governmental cancer centers with 39 linear accelerators (LINACs).

Action 2 calls for expansion of access to radiotherapy targeting at least one cancer center in each LMIC to have radiotherapy services by 2020, and a 25% increase in radiotherapy treatment capacity by 2025. This means 800 to 3000 LINACS are needed for Africa.

Action 3 addresses human resources for radiotherapy, targeting 7500 radiation oncologists, 20 000 radiation technologists, and 6000 medical physicists to be trained in LMICs by 2025. This recognizes that adding machines is only part of the solution. Safe and effective treatment requires trained and knowledgeable physicians. So there must also be access to education and training to build the needed capacity and counter the effects of medical brain drain. This training could be multi-faceted as highlighted in figure 4.2. Currently Varian is actively working to create French and English Educational Hubs in Africa.

Action 4 is a call for funding (finding) the investment to expand access to radiotherapy. Such funding could come from multi-lateral agencies such as the World Bank and development banks. The financing could also come from states

Table 4.1. Lancet Oncology Commission call to action.

Action 1: population-based cancer control plans

- Target: by 2020, 80% of the countries to have cancer plans that include radiotherapy.

Action 2: expansion of access to radiotherapy

- Targets: at least one cancer center in each LMIC by 2020; 25% increase in radiotherapy treatment capacity by 2025.

Action 3: Human resources for radiotherapy

- Target: 7500 radiation oncologists, 20 000 radiation technologists, and 6000 medical physicists to be trained in LMICs by 2025.

Action 4: sustainable financing to expand access to radiotherapy

- Target: $46 billion of investment by 2025 to establish radiotherapy infrastructure and training in LMIC countries.

Action 5: align radiotherapy access with universal health coverage

- Target: 80% of low-income and middle-income countries to include radiotherapy services as part of their universal health coverage by 2020.

THE LANCET Oncology

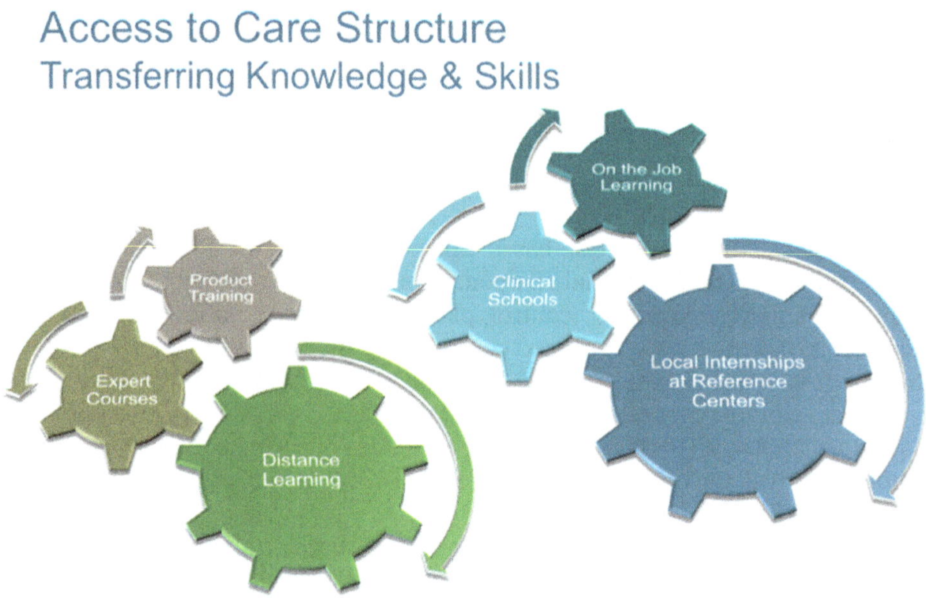

Figure 4.2. The need for capacity building.

(governments), which could be facilitated by export credit agencies, or national aid agencies. Financing could also come from NGOs or charities, via grant funding or vouchers. It could also come from private investors, operators, or suppliers, or a combination of public–private partnerships (PPPs). Overall, over $46 billion is needed by 2025, in investment to establish targeted radiotherapy infrastructure and training in LMICs.

Action 5 calls for LMICs to incorporate radiotherapy as part of universal health coverage, with a target of 80% of LMICs to include radiotherapy as part of universal health coverage by 2020. Here there is an opportunity for both public and private sectors to get involved.

4.1.3 Varian for global radiation oncology

In view of these calls to action, Varian is working towards a future of cancer care technology for quality, efficiency, and cost effectiveness. Varian can

- Provide financial expertise and connections.
- Deliver training and educational programs and people.
- Bring 'leapfrogging' technology to market (see figure 4.3).
- Offer cost effective solutions.
- Advocate at all levels.
- Connect global resources.

By working together the puzzle can be completed. That was how everyone came together to address the growing HIV/Aids epidemic. Today cancer cannot remain the 'silent' killer. Varian's vision is a world without fear of cancer, a partner for life.

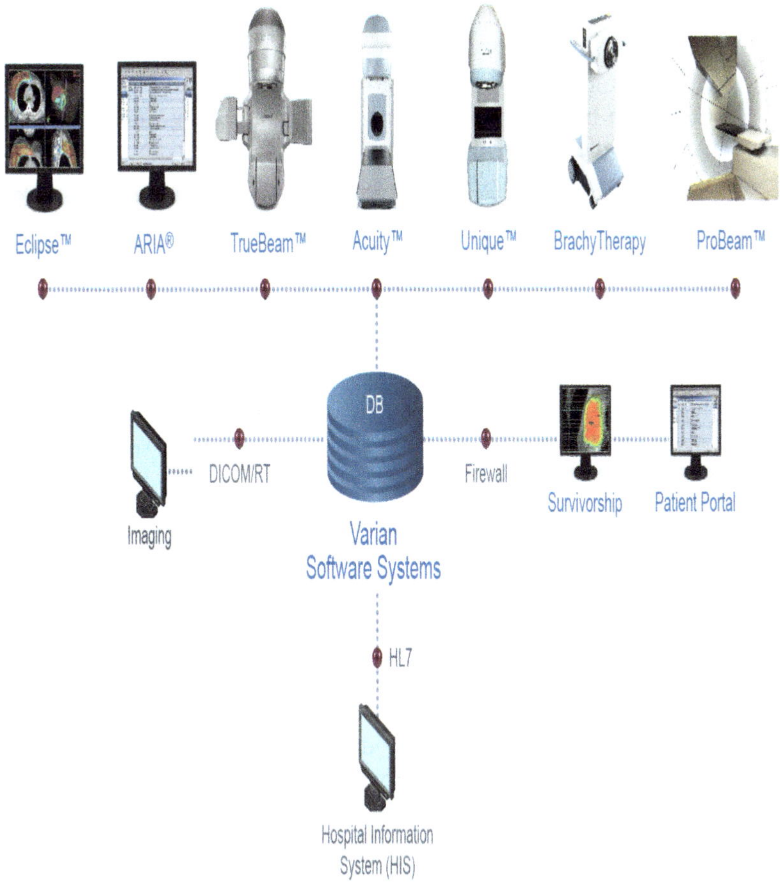

Figure 4.3. The leapfrog potential of new technologies. Reproduced from [2] with permission from IOP Publishing.

4.1.4 Interview questions on the supplier's perspective on sustainable radiotherapy in low resource settings. Interview conducted by Dr Omoruyi Credit Irabor following the lecture by the Varian President

1. Can you detail to us the radiotherapy supply process, and the challenges that are peculiar to low resource countries?
   Answer:
   Challenges:
   - Lack of supportive infrastructure (energy, logistics, etc).
   - Lack of human resources capacity.
   - Cancer plans are often missing or not funded.
   - Lack of financing, combined with no reimbursement models or insurance.
2. What has been the recent trend in the global radiotherapy market and how do you think this has affected or will affect the developing world?
   Answer:
   - Growing awareness of radiotherapy as often the most significant gap in cancer care.

- Growing awareness of total burden of NCDs and cancer on LMICs.
- Continued problems to finance the initial capital investment, and no payment models to cover ongoing coverage costs.
- Interest in innovative solutions (PPPs, financing, market access).

3. So far, what role has your company played in salvaging the disparity in global radiotherapy access? What are the objectives set by your company and how do they intend to achieve these goals? What have been the biggest challenges in meeting these set objectives?
   Answer:
   - Increasing focus on Africa and other LMICs; establishment of education centers these areas.
   - Systematic approaches to priority countries such as Kenya, Nigeria, Uganda, and Tanzania, working with a range of stakeholders and the government to prepare modern comprehensive radiotherapy access strategies.
   - Exploring new payment models for radiotherapy.
4. A novel approach to finding a lasting solution to the gross equipment shortage, first initiated by the IAEA in 2010, was the bid on manufacturers of radiotherapy devices to design equipment packages that are more affordable and suitable for developing countries. How far have the companies gone in pursuit of this technology? And what are the challenges?
   Answer:
   - The majority of radiotherapy design innovation is aimed at treating a larger number of patients more quickly with better clinical outcomes, accompanied by higher reliability and 'uptime'. This is not limited to the developing world but relevant to it, as radiotherapy centers in LMICs can (in principle) operate their machines 2–3 shifts per day, treating up to 60–70 patients per day, and up to 6000 patients per year. Accompanying planning software establishes baseline quality, reduces risk of error, and shortens planning and treatment times further.
   - Ministers and public health decision-makers in LMICs indicate their preference for a range of radiotherapy machines, linked often to a 'hub and spoke' cancer network which higher-end machines clustered in 'hub' academic teaching hospitals. Often they do not want even low energy LINACs, despite the apparent better 'fit' with their environments. As compared to diagnostics—where the benefits of small, mobile diagnostics are clear—it is not certain that LMIC decision-makers favor such development directions.
   - Decision-makers are interested in ways to use available capacity more efficiently—especially when there is unused capacity in private centers—and in reducing the cost per patient treated.
5. In South Africa, several private cancer centers have been established solely through joint ventures with the radiotherapy manufacturers for equipment supply. Yet, this rarely happens in some other countries like Nigeria, which presumably should have a larger market. Why does the technology industry tend to work more with some LMICs than with others? Are there some

unspoken interventions the governments must make? Are there policies that must be enacted to secure a lasting partnership?
Answer:

- It is true that the installed base of linear accelerators in Africa is uneven, with a disproportionate number of machines in South Africa, and in private centers. In some countries, a number of factors have prevented this approach from being taken. They include (1) lack of a well-established private healthcare sector, (2) issues with financing, sovereign guarantees, and investor security, (3) lack of a framework for PPPs, and (4) lack of a plan to leverage the private sector including treating public patients.
- Each government must provide the stable, clear, and predictable market conditions that private investors require. These include sovereign guarantees and operational guarantees to operators; the ability to repatriate capital; and payment models linked to a number of patients treated (increasingly linked to outcomes achieved). To secure a lasting partnership, governments need to work with manufacturers and other stakeholders to determine overall cancer treatment needs and how they can be addressed over time, in a sustainable manner. Expanding coverage over time is a key enabling factor.
- The lack of financing for NCDs—including cancer—remains the biggest single obstacle for all parties in addressing the gap in radiotherapy access in LMICs. Unfortunately, unlike communicable disease, it does not seem likely that any international initiatives—from the UN, private foundations, or Member State governments—will address this gap.

4.2 Conquering cancer

Lecture by Krish Suthanthiran (Founder and President of Best Cure Foundation and TeamBest Group of Companies).

4.2.1 Introduction

My fight against cancer is a personal one. In 1965, my father was diagnosed with colon cancer. Spurred by the death of my father, I have dedicated more than 40 years to cancer research, treatment, and cure—establishing and acquiring a number of medical companies globally in order to collect many of the technologies needed to establish a proactive healthcare delivery system. TeamBest products are used to treat millions of cancer patients globally. On 29 April 2015, in memory of my father and the millions of people affected by cancer, I launched his career-long goal of a 'Global War on Cancer' dedicated to the prevention and cure of cancer.

4.2.2 Global war on cancer

The global war on cancer is envisioned as a proactive healthcare system focused on full transparency of clinical benefits, outcomes, and costs using a total health approach: prevention, early detection, and effective treatment for total cure. It is also focused on making quality healthcare affordable and accessible worldwide using a hub and spoke model of express and mobile healthcare (figure 4.4). In this

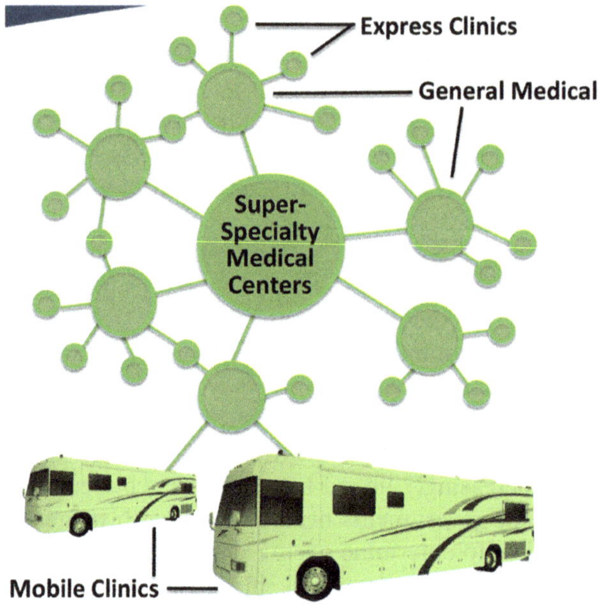

Figure 4.4. Hub and spoke model of healthcare delivery.

approach express and mobile clinics are linked to general and super-specialty medical centers worldwide.

Some of the challenges that must be addressed in the global war against cancer include: corruption, hypocrisy, discrimination of various kinds, dictatorial governing under the name of democracy or dictatorship, and bureaucracy. These add to poor education and healthcare delivery at a very high cost to everyone. I founded my company in 1977 as Best Medical International, Inc. I named it 'Best' because I wanted to be the best in whatever I was doing (figure 4.5). Having acquired many companies and technologies in oncology, cardiology, and radiology, our family of companies has grown and is collectively known as TeamBest.

TeamBest companies manufacture low-tech, medium-tech, high-tech, and highest-to-high-tech products and equipment ranging from \$10 consumable products to \$150 million for a heavy ion particle therapy system. This also covers new novel treatment protocols, devices, multi-center/satellite facilities, and smart spending on solutions so cancer centers and hospitals run effectively.

Cobalt-60 is widely used for conventional radiotherapy in most of the world, which has lacked the required technical research and development to facilitate intensity modulated radiotherapy (IMRT) and image-guided radiotherapy (IGRT), until now. Multi-leaf collimators are now available as an optional accessory for the Equinox and GammaBeam 100-80 product line, providing 3D conformal radiation therapy (3D CRT) and IMRT capability. TeamBest products have proven reliability with over 45 000 treatments performed worldwide every day. Some centers treat 100+ patients/day with over 3000 installations worldwide, which are cost-effective, with lower infrastructure and energy demands, and reduced quality assurance and staff demands—as well as lower maintenance fees

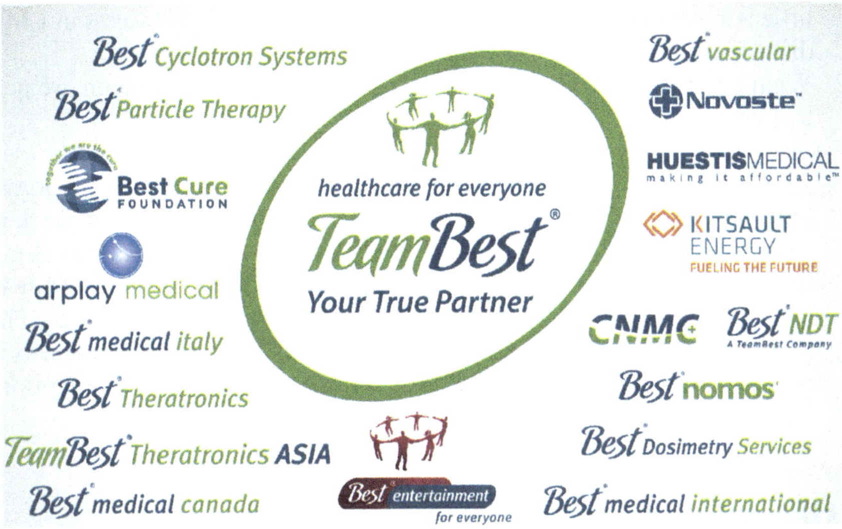

Figure 4.5. TeamBest companies. Reproduced with permission from [4].

4.2.3 Best Cure Foundation

There is an Indian proverb that says that 'a healthy person has many wishes, but a sick person has only one'. The Best Cure Foundation's mission is to keep the healthy person healthy. And should someone get sick, the goal is early detection, effective treatment, and total cure. The Best Cure Foundation goals can be summarized as:

- Providing purified drinking water and affordable sewer systems in every part of the world.
- Promoting our division 3E (Triple E)—Education, Empowerment, and Equality—to promote everyone regardless of ethnicity and gender, by treating all as equals
- Significantly reducing suffering and death due to cancer, cardiac disease, diabetes, and contagious diseases.

Please join me in this global war on cancer: www.bestcure.md, www.teambest.com

4.2.4 Interview questions on the supplier's perspective to sustainable radiotherapy in low resource settings. Interview conducted by Dr Credit Omoruyi following the lecture by the TeamBest President.

1. What role can a radiotherapy manufacturer play in global health?
   Answer:
   How much more can we achieve with more precise radio-therapeutics in comparison to wider radiotherapy access? We have saved human lives with scientific advances in radiation medicine; however, the number dwindles if compared to that saved by an increment in access. 70% of cancer mortalities now occur in LMICs with no access to our many advances, thus, seeing how

little is spent in ensuring cancer prevention and treatment access in LMICs is disturbing. It is time to make global health a priority

2. What challenges in radiotherapy management and supply-chain are peculiar to LMICs?

   Answer:

   I am afraid that the decision to adopt one radiotherapy technology over another in LMICs is currently being made on the grounds of market and self-interest rather than on sustainability or suitability. This bias is evident in the current reimbursement system for LINAC over cobalt, in spite of the higher longevity and lower maintenance costs for cobalt machines. There is also a need for public enlightenment in LMICs, not only with regards to the prevention and treatment of cancer, but also of the public corruption that has impeded progress in cancer care

4.3 Global Oncology (GO)

Lecture by Franklin Huang (Co-Founder and Co-President Global Oncology, http://globalonc.org/).

4.3.1 Introduction

Global Oncology (GO) is a non-profit organization dedicated to bringing the best in cancer care to underserved patients around the world. GO's unique volunteer network of professionals drawn from medicine, science, engineering, design, and public health backgrounds work in teams to help people throughout the world who are treating cancer and its related pain.

GO projects are developed and run by highly skilled volunteers and are mentored by senior volunteers. Current programs and projects are in the areas of advanced training, education, and technology development. GO collaborates with international partners to improve cancer care, research, and education in resource-limited settings.

Cancer patients in low income countries may lack knowledge of their diagnosis and what to expect with treatment, and have low literacy rates. GO's first-of-its-kind Cancer Educational Materials (CEM) are designed for low-literacy patients in

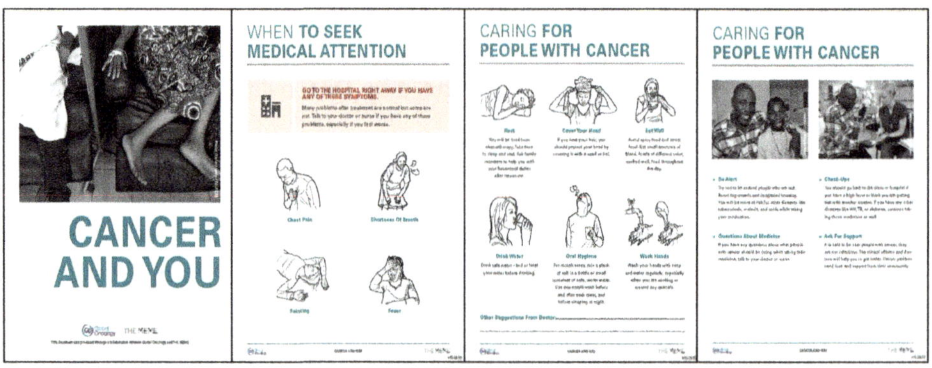

Figure 4.6. GO Cancer educational materials. Reproduced with permission from [4].

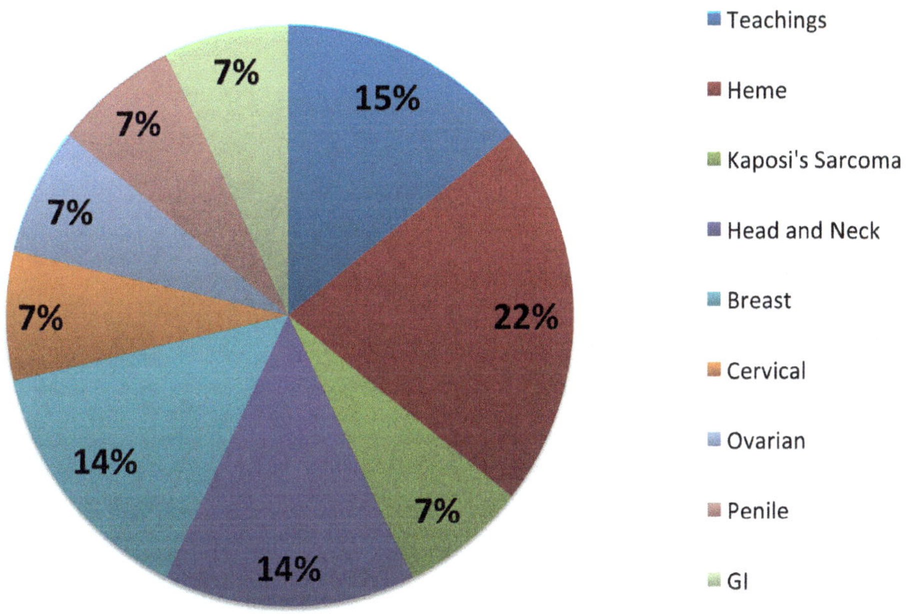

Figure 4.7. Tumor boards by numbers. Reproduced with permission from [5].

resource-limited settings to illustrate the side-effects of cancer treatments and recommendations on the care of cancer patients. Importantly, these materials were co-created and designed with input and feedback from care providers and patients in Malawi, Rwanda, and Haiti. GO CEM pilot sites include: Queen Elizabeth Central Hospital Blantyre, Malawi; Butaro Cancer Center of Excellence, Rwanda; and Hospital Mirebelais, Haiti.

4.3.2 GO-QECH case conferences and tumor boards

GO-QECH Case Conferences are a forum to advise on difficult cancer cases. With only one oncologist, complex cancer cases in Malawi lack specialized oncology expertise. GO established a collaboration with Dr Leo Masamba at Queen Elizabeth Central Hospital (QECH) to develop a tumor board/case conference to provide consultation and teaching on complex cancer cases presenting to the cancer ward at QECH. The GO-QECH Tumor Board Collaboration was established in February 2013 with goal to improve the care of cancer patients in Malawi through knowledge-sharing, mentoring, and education. Oncologists based in Boston consult and teach on complex cancer cases presented by colleagues in Malawi.

4.3.3 Global Cancer Project Map (theGOMap.org)

More than ever before, NGOs, academia, government, and industry are making efforts to improve cancer control. However, it has been nearly impossible to efficiently figure out who is doing what and where. Collaboration can stall and be

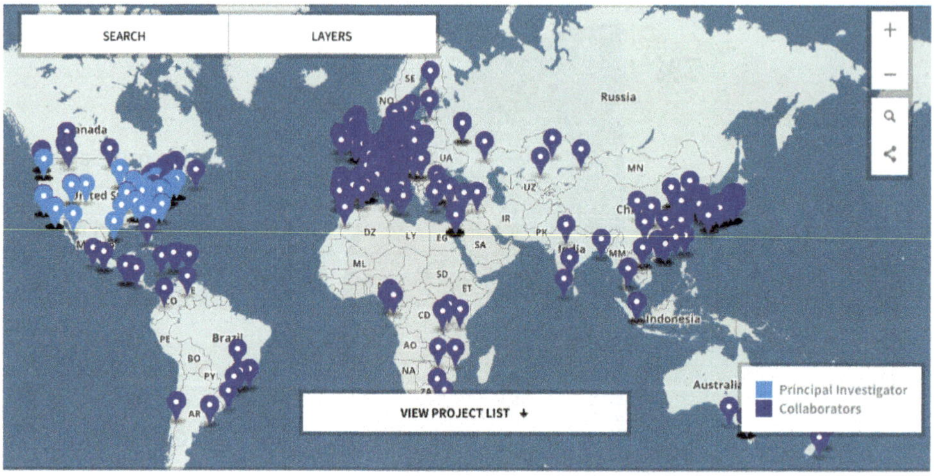

Figure 4.8. GO map on global cancer research. Reproduced with permssion from [6].

difficult due to lack of knowledge of ongoing and previous work in specific countries or areas. The GO Map (thegomap.org) was designed to address this problem. It is the single largest worldwide geospatial database of cancer research, training, and control projects (figure 4.8). It was developed to catalyze and enable communication, collaboration, and partnerships in the global oncology community, identify information and research gaps, and prevent duplication of efforts that waste limited resources. The map was co-founded and produced by NCI/CGH and Global Oncology, Inc., in partnership with the Union for International Cancer Control (UICC) and the American Society for Clinical Oncology (ASCO).

The map allows for visualizing of networks of cancer projects, using data to guide cancer control efforts. This includes: cancer research (basic science), cancer care (clinical), cancer control and screening (public health), and capacity building. Search options include: by project type, by country, by 29 World Health Organization cancer types, by organization name or type, by funding source, by project start and end dates, and by keywords. Projects can be submitted to the GO Map as well.

In summary, the GO Map was first released on 25 March 2015 as a web-based platform that catalogs international cancer research, cancer care, and cancer outreach programs. The newest release of the GO Map will occur in 2017 and will include networking and improved data features. The platform aims to align cancer care efforts of governmental agencies, non-profit organizations, academic institutions and industry partners. The GCPM's primary objectives are to:

1. Facilitate the breaking down of silos and building of collaboration.
2. Accelerate progress, ensure a balanced investment of resources, and align global cancer care and cancer efforts.
3. Provide a simple way to visualize international efforts in cancer research and control.

4.4 Need for global radiation oncology care collaborations: example, Cameroon

Lecture presented by Samba Richard (Special Radiation Protection Projects Coordinator, International Atomic Energy Agency (IAEA) NRPA, Cameroon).

4.4.1 Introduction

Cameroon is widely referred to as 'Africa in miniature'. It is located on a strategic shipping route in Africa. There is political stability to encourage foreign investment and the country provides a window for import/export/transit of goods to neighboring central African countries. The top five cancers for both sexes in Yaoundé, the capital of Cameroon, are shown in table 4.2. These are likely under-reported due to poor cancer registries.

Breast and cervical cancers account for more than half of cancers among women, while prostate and liver comprise more than a third of cancers for men. Cancer is of significant public health concern and its treatment poses a problem. Cameroon has cancer centers only in Yaoundé General Hospital and Douala General Hospital. However, at present, only Douala has a functional radiotherapy facility. Two teletherapy Co-60 machines and a brachytherapy system are available in Douala. Most patients undergoing radiotherapy are treated with external beam radiotherapy (EBRT). EBRT is delivered alone or in combination with brachytherapy. Many cancer patients treated with EBRT also receive concomitant chemotherapy. Only 16% of the cancer patients in Cameroon receive radiotherapy, mainly for two reasons: the high cost of radiotherapy treatment and a shortage of radiotherapy facilities in the country.

Constraints in patients' access to cancer treatment (radiotherapy, chemotherapy, and surgical services) presents a significant challenge for Cameroon's cancer control program. The regulatory body (National Radiation Protection Agency (NRPA)) has been mandated through laws and regulations to regulate all ionizing radiation

Table 4.2. Top five cancers (both sexes) in Yaoundé.

	Number of cases						
Cancer	2004	2005	2006	2010	2011	Total	Ages standardized rate per 100 000
Breast (women)	177	157	175	165	163	837	35.2
Cervix	110	132	145	135	129	651	27.7
Lymphomas (both)	96	*	79	60	*	559	17.2
Prostate	77	78	105	28	54	342	16.7
Kaposi	46	95	89	49	40	319	10.7 (men) 4.1 (women)
All types	970	1096	1071	756	784	4689	44.3 (men) 62.3 (women)

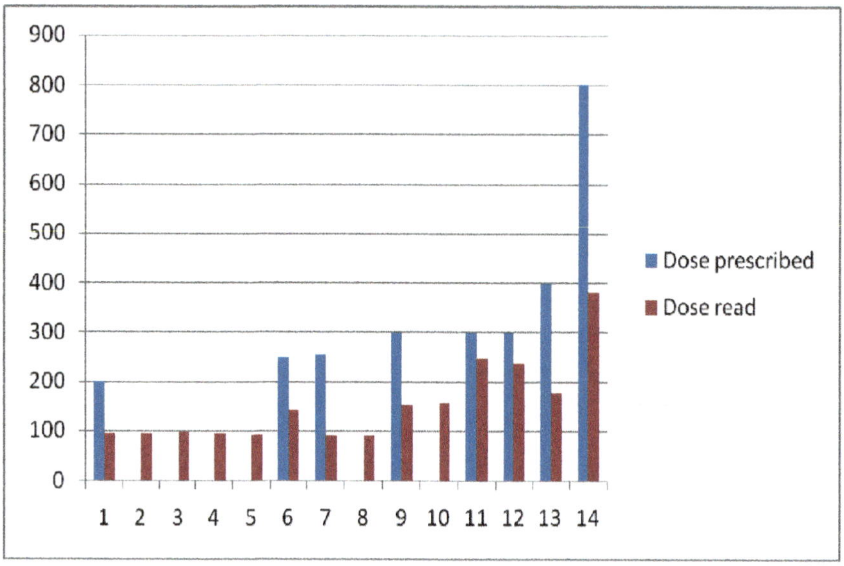

Figure 4.9. Dose of patient audit using OSL nanodots.

sources as well as the protection of people and environment against ionizing radiation hazards. There are only three certified Medical Physicists with one working with the NRPA. It is hoped that with the collaboration and help of renowned medical physics associations, the International Atomic Energy Agency (IAEA), the World Health Organization (WHO), and non-profit organizations, together with the Cameroon Ministry of Public Health, Scientific Research and Higher Education, the fight against cancer will be taken to a new improved level through global collaboration and modern technology.

4.4.2 Treatment planning and delivery

Treatment simulation was performed by oncologists without a treatment planning system (TPS). Optically stimulated luminescence (OSL) nanodots were used for dose audit absorbed by the skin of the patients. Calibration was needed before reading the nanodots for radiation oncology patient monitoring, since the reader was previously calibrated only for individual monitoring. Sample results are shown in figure 4.9. It was found that the doses prescribed were higher than the doses delivered with a variant of about 80%. This is alarming and highlights a major problem in African LMICs, where apparently there is significant under-dosing or overdosing when using poor radiation medicine technologies.

4.4.3 Recommendations/perspective

Consistent with the Lancet Oncology Commission report, there is great need to establish a national radiotherapy plan covering the medium and long term. There is a need to increase radiotherapy capacity in the short term at the two existing centers

(Yaoundé and Douala) by addressing all relevant areas (staffing, equipment, quality assurance programs, and maintenance policy). There is also the need to perform regular quality control of equipment and ensure regular maintenance and servicing, and to standardize treatment protocols for the most common cancers.

Leaders, governments, private sector, and non-governmental organizations need to be lobbied to take the necessary action so that we can address the growing cancer burden. Education and training programs should accompany the general policy of cancer management. All relevant specialty programs in medical and non-medical fields should be initiated at local universities to provide the required human resources. Increasing the capacity for cancer diagnosis in the areas of pathology, radiology, and nuclear medicine by ensuring availability of qualified human resources (professionals and technicians) and appropriate equipment (echography, mammography, CT scan and MRI) is greatly needed.

Also there is great need to establish adequate radiation protection measures for personnel and patients, in particular in the brachytherapy unit of the Douala General Hospital, in compliance with national legislation and conditions imposed by the regulatory body, and take necessary actions to ensure that all radiology, radiotherapy, and nuclear medicine departments in Cameroon have a valid license issued by the NRPA.

In palliative care there is also a need to revise the current legislation on opioids to cover opioid supply, storage, and prescription. It is necessary to establish a list of essential medicines for palliative care (including oral preparations of morphine and other essential analgesics) in line with the WHO Essential Medicines in Palliative Care.

While the need for collaborations has been expressed for the case of Cameroon, most African countries face similar challenges, with some not even having any radiotherapy facilities. For countries that have radiation medicine technologies, the issue of radiation protection and safety is a big concern that needs to be addressed or emphasized, along with the Lancet Oncology commission calls for action.

4.5 The pain divide: palliative care

Lecture presented by Dr Christian Ntizimira, (Palliative Care Expert and Educator, Rwanda Palliative Care and Hospice Organization; Researcher Collaborator, Lancet Commission of Global Access to Palliative Care & Pain Control). Includes background content from Dr Ntizimira's opinion article at eHospice.

The following is an excerpt from an article by the author, first published by eHospice [7].

> It was in March 2014, during my outpatient consultation at Kibagabaga Hospital in Kigali, that I met my new patient Iganbire (her name has been changed for confidentiality), a vibrant young lady, aged 25 with big eyes and a wonderful smile. As with many young Rwandan women, wearing make-up, lipstick and slim fitted clothes have become commonplace fashion adopted by

this new young generation, influenced by top model mannequins observed through the media.

When I saw her entering the outpatient office, I assumed she came as a caregiver of one of her parents or on behalf of one of the patients we had in the community. However, to my surprise, the nurse I worked with handed me Iganbire's patient file.

'Good morning doctor,' she said articulately in her mother tongue Kinyarwanda, accompanied by a radiant smile.

'Good Morning Ingabire, how are you?' I replied.

'I'm fine but I've had chest pain since last week,' she said. As she spoke, her gaze descended and the volume of her voice diminished.

'I have been referred to you by the surgeon from the Rwanda Military Hospital for pain management because I had been diagnosed with cancer on the left breast two years ago, which was treated with a mastectomy and chemotherapy. Last year, I felt small nodules in my right breast and returned to my surgeon, who suspected the cancer may have returned to my other breast.'

It was clear that underneath all Iganbire's external exhibition of style, that this young woman was psychologically devastated by the diagnosis. I was surprised to see she came alone, without any person to accompany her especially during this difficult time.

'Has someone come with you like your parents, uncle or aunt?' I asked her.

'Unfortunately not!' she said.

'Why? Are they busy? Because I need to talk to your family about the way forward,' I replied.

She then told me with all her large brown eyes widened further, 'All my family died during the genocide against the Tutsis in 1994…I lived with a family friend which was a neighbor prior the genocide. I have no parents, uncles, aunts, even cousins; all of them have been killed during the genocide. I'm alone,' she finished saying with tears in her eyes.

I got goose bumps when she answered my questions and also felt guilty for not being able to help her as I had wished. With tears and a handkerchief in her hand, she added, 'if my mother was here, [maybe] none of this would have happened, I wish I could have died with her during the genocide.' Those words were like a sword pierced into my heart.

Ingabire was five years old when the Genocide against the Tutsi started. At the time, she was living in Kigali with her parents, two elder brothers and two sisters. Her last image of her parents was when her mom took and hid her in a small place behind a house. Soldiers from the Rwanda Patriotic Front found her two days later, weak with fear.

Significance of the memorial week

Ingabire is among the million people in Rwanda who survived the Genocide against the Tutsi in 1994. During the week from April 7 to 14, 2015, Rwanda commemorated 21 years since the genocide.

Every year, during this memorial week, public hospitals are prepared to receive many cases with trauma disorders, which emerge during the commemoration: crying, convulsion, screaming, and loss of conscience. At the same time we have to face a double challenge from patients who survived the genocide and are living with chronic or life limiting diseases.

As a palliative care doctor, I daily experience the ramifications of working in a post-genocide society and its impact on patients and caregivers facing life-threatening illness. I've learnt to manage these cases at a different level compared to cases of patients who are not genocide survivors. Case management should indeed be different because of the patient's background and experiences, the context of the disease and psychological impact.

In their article Rieder and Elbert, *Conflict and Health* (2013) [1], discuss the Post Traumatic Syndrome Disorders (PTSD), mental health and psychological problems of survivors, former prisoners and their children following a period marked with neighbors attacking neighbors with 'guns, machetes or sticks,' looting, destruction of property, and 'genocidal acts including murder and sexual violence.'

Rieder and Elbert continue to note how '...entire family systems as well as the general social fabric that formerly provided support were destroyed due to losses of family members and growing mistrust and fear following the genocide.'

Patient autonomy in a post genocide context

In the Rwandan context, the cultural impact is important and I have learned to work with respect to the culture, while combining modern management principles to improve the quality of life of my patients.

Iganbire's context in relation to patient autonomy is best described in the saying, 'When you are well you belong to yourself, but when you are sick you belong to your family.' As long as someone is well, they have the autonomy to make their own decisions, their own plan and decide about their own future. However, as soon as that person becomes sick, especially with a chronic disease, even if they are still able to make some decisions, it's automatically the family's decision that orients the patient management of care.

Since I've started work in palliative care in Rwanda, I have never been contacted by the patient himself or herself, even if they were able to do so. It's always been the members of the patient's family calling me for an appointment for their loved one to explain the patient's treatment history, expectations and to discuss their future plan of management.

In Western countries, patient autonomy is really clear and the implications of family engagement will depend most of the time on the patient's decision, which is to be respected. However, when I recently discussed the concept of culture impact versus patient autonomy with a palliative physician colleague from the United States, she shared that in her context 'when you are well you belong to yourself but when you are sick you belong to your home.'

Palliative care as an Ubuntu approach

The WHO defines palliative care as 'an approach.' In my opinion, as an African and palliative physician, the definition of palliative care is beyond an 'approach', it's a concept which encompasses an 'Ubuntu philosophy' defined as 'I am what I am because of who we all are.' Or, 'I am a person through other persons.' It speaks particularly about the fact that you can't exist as a human being in isolation. It speaks about our interconnectedness.

The patient is not a single component of him/herself or a single unit of input into data, but a component interconnected with the other as a person, a father, a mother, sibling, a member of a community, society, a country, and continent. Back to the Rwandan context, I've learnt three lessons from my experiences in palliative care in a humanitarian context in dealing with survivor patients:

History and background matter: The first and most important lesson when you want to manage the care of survivor patients from massive traumatic situations is to understand their history, not only their stories. Pain management and palliative care for patients in humanitarian contexts should be treated differently compared to the same patients with the same diagnosis with a different context. The patient's history and background must be accounted for. Why? During the period of commemoration, for example, patients developed more psychosocial pain than physical pain. Whatever the quantity of strong opioids that may be used, they still feel pain. The WHO ladder doesn't work in such a context. Another pain management approach is needed to address the patient's history and background. For example, a patient impacted by a mass traumatic situation like a tsunami, civil war, Ebola, genocide, rape, in the diagnosis and treatment of cancer will react differently in their management compared to a patient who has never been affected by these situations.

The psychological context of disease: As a physician, I could explain easily the physiopathology of diseases then decide on the best course of treatment. For most of my patients who survived the genocide, chronic diseases or life-limiting illnesses are considered as a punishment or a consequence of genocide. In my previous eHospice article on 'Providing palliative care in post genocide Rwanda,' I explained that 'a lot of patients express during counseling that they feel that there is a strong correlation between what happened to them during the genocide and their current situation.' Patients identify themselves with the disease as a consequence of a post genocide situation, or an instrument of identification to those who died during the genocide. With these patients, I have to use different language, ridden with compassion as a person rather than a physician, explaining in simple language about their disease. One of my strategies when I'm visiting these patients is to remove my lab coat to break the barrier between the physician-to-patient pedestal to empathize at the patient and family member's level, especially for a lethal diagnosis.

Correlation between survivor patients and social support: In Rwanda, the psychosocial aspects of palliative care must be given great focus as so many were affected by the genocide. If we avoid this reality then one fails to offer effective palliative care. As a physician I must consider: how deeply this situation has affected my patients? How is the patient able to cope with his/her loss? In our cultural context, because someone who is sick belongs to their family, the best way to manage the patient's psychological problems is to support families and caregivers. It took time during my practice to understand the strong relation between patients and family, sometimes I took both of them as one unit. However, there is a strong correlation between family psychology behavior and patient psychological impact, and one can affect the other and vice versa. Research into the psychological impact of survivor patients with cancer or incurable diseases in the context of palliative care could help us to understand the scope of this correlation.

During the genocide, a part of our humanity was lost along with the one million who perished. However, I'm still convinced that the concept of palliative care will bring back this part of humanity lost and will teach us to understand the deep perception of being a 'human being' in extending hope for the Rwandan post genocide society.

—Christian Ntizimira

4.5.1 Introduction

During the Rwandan Genocide in 2004, ca 1 000 000 people were killed during 100 days, resulting in a million refugees. Post traumatic syndrome disorders (PTSD) in Rwandan society are prevalent as a consequence, and mental health is a huge issue to solve [7, 8].

Palliative care is an approach that improves the quality of life of patients and their families facing the problems associated with life-threatening illness, through the prevention and relief of suffering by means of early identification and impeccable assessment and treatment of pain and other problems, physical, psychosocial, and spiritual [9].

4.5.2 Palliative care in Rwanda

Documented cases show that around 15 800 patients (HIV + cancers) died with moderate and severe pain from 2007 to 2009 [10]. The estimation of patients who suffered from pain was greater than 85%. This situation reflects what Felicia Knaul *et al* characterize as the global pain divide and the great need for collaborations to close the global cancer/pain divide [11] (figure 4.10). The World Health Organization estimates that every year tens of millions of people, including 5.5 million terminal cancer patients, suffer needlessly in severe pain because they do not have access to pain medications. A recent study found that more than four out of every five people on the planet live in countries with low to non-existent access to opioids for pain [4].

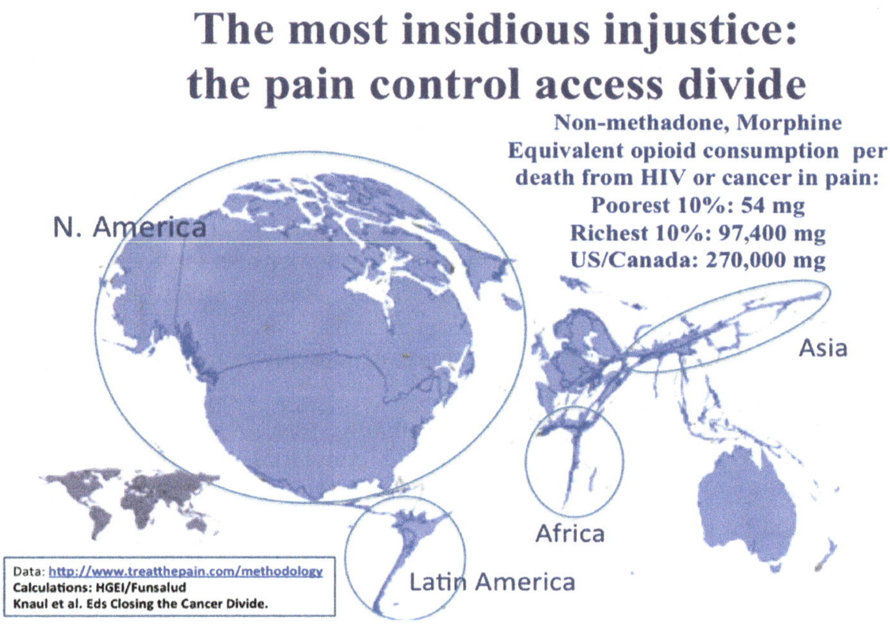

Figure 4.10. The global pain divide. Reproduced with permission from [11].

Before palliative care came to Rwanda, a large number of cancer patients suffered from severe pain in the hospital. The example of Kibagabaga Hospital, a large district hospital city of Kigali, has shown that the morphine used was less than 4%, with a bed occupancy rate of 120%, non-existent psychosocial support, and more than 89% of the patients died with moderate and severe pain. There was also opiophobia, 'fear of opioids'. The protocol was prohibitive involving, Red Ink + three signatures for one ampule of morphine. There was also often conflict between pharmacists, MDs, and anesthetists, and there was no linkage of continuum care at the community level.

4.5.3 Interventions

Key components for intervention include:

- Multidisciplinary palliative care teams within treatment facilities.
- Integration of palliative care to the community level.
- Structured training.
- Introduction of the Ubuntu philosophy: 'A person is a person through other people'.

In 2005 the Rwanda Minister of Health invited Partners in Health to help expand healthcare access in rural Rwanda. In 2011 the Butaro Hospital was inaugurated and in July 2012 the Butaro Cancer Center of Excellence (BCCOE) was inaugurated. Many patients continue to benefit from this center. The prevailing challenges include: turnover of personnel trained; training in palliative care for children;

palliative care needs for others; curriculum of palliative care not yet integrated in the School of Health Sciences; the importance of 'Stoicism' as an important cultural value; little research; and mental health issues among palliative care patients, which may still be attributed to the genocide.

4.5.4 Conclusion

Palliative care is not optional. It is not an extra, an addition, a luxury, or an afterthought. It is an essential component of humane cancer care. To develop cancer treatments without parallel development of palliative care is a cruel injustice to the millions of cancer patients around the world who suffer needlessly. In every country, it is absolutely essential that when people talk about access to radiotherapy and cervical cancer screening and chemotherapy—all vitally important—they must also be talking in equal measure and with equal conviction about access to palliative care.

Acknowledgements

The author is grateful to the Rwanda Ministry of Health, the Rwanda Palliative Care and Hospice Organization, the Lancet Commission on access to Palliative Care and Pain Control, Dr Wilfred Ngwa, and Dr Eric Krakauer.

4.6 The Global Health Catalyst Win–Win Initiative

Lecture by Ahmed Elzawawy (President of ICEDOC) and Esther Ikiara (CEO, Mombasa Cancer Care Center Kenya).

4.6.1 Introduction

In December 2007, The Win–Win Scientific initiative was proposed by Ahmed Elzawawy as an initiative of ICEDOC's Experts in Cancer Without Borders www.icedoc.org/winwin.htm. It aims at increasing the availability of better value cancer treatment in the world via exploring scientific approaches. All the stakeholders—particularly cancer patients and their families—can win. This also includes helping the business of pharmaceutical companies and manufacturers of radiotherapy machines and medical devices to flourish without ruining a country's or individual's economy.

There are two mains wings of the Win–Win Initiative. The first wing is 'Exploring scientific approaches to increase affordability of better value cancer care'. The second wing of the Win–Win Initiative was proposed in November 2015 and declared on 29 April 2016 during the Harvard Global Health Catalyst (GHC) summit. This wing focuses on catalyst action and professional advice to increase enormously the rate of establishment of services of clinical oncology in the world, starting with the most difficult challenges in Africa.

On 29 April 2016, the Win–Win Initiative joined the Harvard GHC and became one of its activities. Leaders of the Win–Win Initiative, such as Professor Elzawawy,

Table 4.3. Costs estimates for MCCC.

Capital expenditure	Phase 1 & 2 Partial	
Non-current assets	Cost KSHS	Cost USD
LAND	25 000 000	250 000
BUNKER	33 000 000	330 000
FACILITY BUILDING	110 000 000	1 100 000
FACILITY EQUIPMENT		
Linat Accel erator		
Ultrasound	10 000 000	100 000
CT Scan	70 000 000	700 000
Brachtherapy	20 000 000	200 000
Mammogram	18 000 000	130 000
Oxygen Generating Plant	15 000 000	150 000
Ambulance	5 000 000	50 000
Shipping cost	5 000 000	50 000
Minor Theatre Equipment	2 000 000	20 000
Installation costs	5 000 000	50 000
Lab Equipment	6 000 000	60 000
	324 000 000	3 240 000
OTHER EQUIPMENT		
Generator	3 000 000	30 000
Server & Computers	2 000 000	20 000
Air Conditioners	600 000	6000
Bed & Lockers	2 000 000	20 000
Bell System	300 000	3000
CCTV	500 000	5000
Hospital Furniture	2 000 000	20 000
TV sets	400 000	4000
Chemotherapy Reclining Chairs	750 000	7500
Laundry Machine	120 000	1200
Fridges	200 000	2000
Kitchen Equipment	1 500 000	15 000
	13 370 000	133 700
Total Capital Expenditure	337 370 000	3 373 700

Notes:

The cost of facility building and bunker is an estimation provided by the project's architect.

The LINAC accelerator cost will not be included in the capital expenditure budget as the machine has been donated.

All equipment costs have been pegged at current market prices are professional consultants and volunteer catalysts. So, as facilitators, they are encouraging everyone to connect and to communicate with each other and to collaborate or partner. The Win–Win Initiative is not meant to compete with or replace any society, organization, body, governmental or private efforts, or individuals.

During the 2016 summit, the Win–Win session brought together industry leaders with stakeholders from LMICs to catalyze the establishment or expansion of cancer centers that can become hubs of excellence in LMICs. One of the projects presented was the Mombasa Cancer Care Center in Kenya.

4.6.2 The Mombasa Cancer Care Center, Kenya: proposed project

The Mombasa Cancer Care Center (2016–2021) is an example of a project by LMIC stake-holders looking to establish a cancer center in their country. The mission of the Mombasa Cancer Care Center is to offer accessible, affordable, subsidized and/or free comprehensive cancer management to all, regardless of their status. The project, proposed during the 2016 GHC summit, will be situated on the north coast of Mombasa/Kilifi County. The plan involved acquiring 1.5 acres of land on the Malindi Highway for ease of access for all patients; either by public means or private vehicles.

4.6.2.1 Project roadmap

The aim is to set up a center that will offer a comprehensive approach, from health education, prevention, screening, treatment, training, and research, as well as a hospice, within a period of approximately five years (by 2021) depending on availability of resources. The first phase will mainly offer outreach, awareness, screening, diagnostic, radiation, chemotherapy, minor surgeries, and day care services. The second phase should flag in a major theatre, recovery ward, training, and research as well as a hospice.

The third phase should then incorporate high dose chemotherapy with a stem cell transplant unit and any other related treatment towards alleviating the patient's plight.

4.6.2.2 Achievements

A Varian high energy 18 MV radiotherapy machine has been generously donated by James Shakey, Senior Vice President of Oncology Services International (OSI). Also, the company Cyber deem, through Mr Helmy Ayman, is willing to carry out installation of the machine after the bunker is constructed, with reasonable fees. Guidelines for the construction of the bunker have already been issued.

Professor Elzawawy (President of ICEDOC) and a team of professionals are providing support, with some willing to offer free services to needy patients. The Mombasa Cancer Care Center (MCCC) has been incorporated into an existing non-governmental Cancer Research and Communication Organization (CRCO).

A volunteer team comprising technical, administrative, and finance people was formed, and has been working hard to come up with a comprehensive tentative project proposal.

4.6.2.3 Cost of establishment

The tentative project establishment costs are shown in table 4.3 for phase 1. The facility can be constructed in different stages depending on the funding, with the immediate needs being the bunker, and absolutely necessary areas.

The current appeal is supported in many ways, from well-wishers, donors, and partners both local and international, to help actualize this noble service to save the lives of many who are suffering and eventually dying due to various factors including, but not limited to: late detection, lack of adequate affordable services, and lack of adequate facilities to reach the people in their locality (currently all the above services are in the capital city Nairobi). We have only a few professionals, who are unable to cater for the huge number of patients, etc.

We also humbly appeal for funding for the cost of initial establishment, so that we are able to offer affordable services to all who require it. A plan for sustainability has been proposed in our detailed projections.

Our desire is that with small steps taken progressively, we shall one day be able to offer these services at very minimal costs/highly subsidized, or better still have many deserving patients access these services free of charge. This is already the case for some communicable diseases (HIV, TB) which have attained free programs for the needy as they receive heavy funding from many donors and government subsidies.

4.6.2.4 Example outcomes of the Win–Win Initiative

Some of the outcomes from the 2016 Win–Win Initiative included the development of a roadmap to establish the cancer center in Mombasa and a roadmap for the establishment of a radiotherapy facility at Mbingo in Cameroon. The projects now both have LINACs and support for education and training, and a concrete plan to realize the project.

Building on this progress, in 2017 the GHC is scaling this up, catalyzing win–win partnerships/support working with industry players such as Varian, TeamBest, etc, non-profit organizations such as Global Oncology, International Agencies such as the IAEA, and LMIC institution stake-holders. There is a growing list of LMIC institutions, including: Tanzania, Rwanda, Nigeria, South Africa, Kenya, Cameroon, Democratic Republic of Congo, Namibia, and Ivory Coast. This tradition should grow in upcoming years until all LMICs in Africa have a viable cancer center to meet the 2022 goal, helping save lives and reduce global cancer disparities.

References

[1] Atun R *et al* 2015 Expanding global access to radiotherapy *The Lancet Oncol.* **16** 1153–86

[2] Ngwa W and Ngoma T 2016 *Emerging Models for Global Health in Radiation Oncology* (Bristol: IOP Publishing)

[3] TeamBest Companies www.teambest.com

[4] Cancer Education Materials—Global Oncology Initiative (GO!) http://globalonc.org/Projects/patient-education-materials/ Accessed June 21, 2017

[5] Partners In Health 2013 The Butaro Cancer Center at One Year www.pih.org/blog/treating-cancer-in-rwanda-the-butaro-cancer-center-at-one-year Accessed June 21, 2017

[6] The GO Map—Global Oncology Initiative (GO!) http://globalonc.org/Projects/global-cancer-project-map/ Accessed June 21, 2017

[7] Ntizimira C 2013 Integration of palliative care in Rwanda (Ehospice) www.ehospice.com/africa/Default/tabid/10701/ArticleId/5401 Accessed June 21, 2017

[8] Rieder H and Elbert T 2013 Rwanda—lasting imprints of a genocide: trauma, mental health and psychosocial conditions in survivors, former prisoners and their children *Conflict Health* **7** 6

[9] World Health Organization 2012 WHO Definition of Palliative Care www.who.int/cancer/palliative/definition/en/ Accessed June 21, 2017

[10] Lohman D, Schleifer R and Amon J J 2010 Access to pain treatment as a human right *BMC Med.* **8** 8

[11] Knaul F M *et al* 2012 *Closing the Cancer Divide: An Equity Imperative* (Cambridge, MA: Harvard University Press) chapter 1 http://isites.harvard.edu/fs/docs/icb.topic1159768.files/CCD_Book_Chapter_1.pdf Accessed March 17, 2017

Chapter 5

Global oncology outreach: cancer prevention and advocacy

Seun Adebiyi, Ophira Ginsburg, Marc Williams, Terence Ngwa, Lydia Asana and Kenneth Ngwa

5.1 Closing the cancer divide: best buys in prevention and advocacy

Lecture by Seun Adebiyi, Esq. (Project Manager for Global Health, American Cancer Society); co-edited by Wilfred Ngwa.

This lecture will cover:

- Drivers of disparity in cancer burden between poor and rich countries.
- 'Best buys' in prevention: taxing tobacco and the HPV vaccine.
- 'Best buys' in advocacy: evidence-based grassroots movement, youth empowerment.

5.1.1 Drivers of disparity in cancer burden

Cancer was once considered a 'Western' disease, only affecting people in the developed world in Europe and America. Today, we know that cancer is a growing healthcare crisis and a major burden for both high income countries (HICs) and low and middle income countries (LMICs). However, the occurrence of cancer looks different in lower income countries (figure 5.1). In terms of epidemiology, of the worlds' 7.1 billion population, 1.3 billion are in more developed countries with 5.8 billion (82%) in developing countries. The recent World Health Organization report puts the incidence of cancer at about 14.1 million new cases a year, with 8 million (57%) of those in less developed countries. Of the 8.2 million deaths a year, 5.3 million (65%) are in less developed countries. The risk of getting cancer by age 75 in is 19% globally, 27% in more developed countries, and 15% in less developed countries. Meanwhile, the risk of dying of cancer by age 75 is 10% globally, 11% in more developed countries, and 10% in less developed countries. While cancer incidence levels off in the US, it is increasing in less developed countries due to aging populations, adoption of a Western lifestyle, and high incidence of infection-related

doi:10.1088/978-0-7503-1359-9ch5

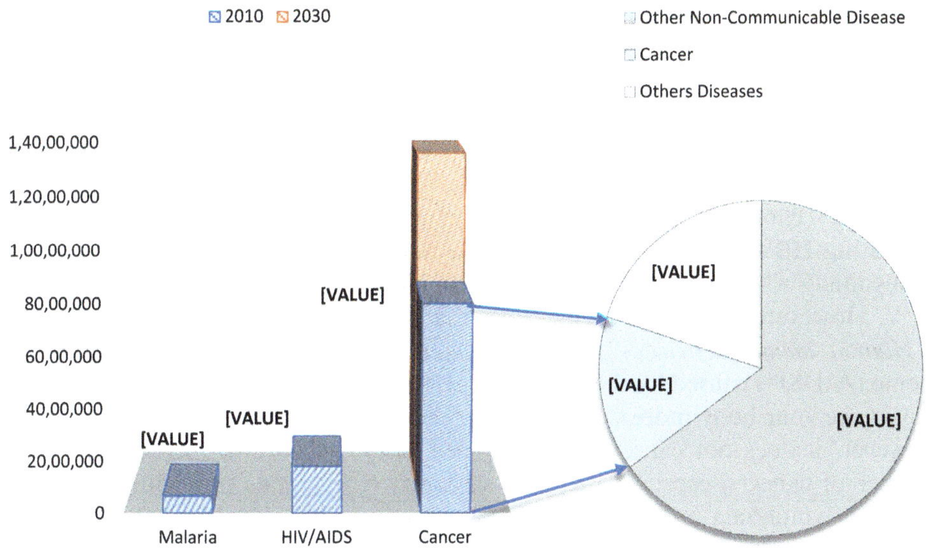

Figure 5.1. Global cancer burden.

cancers, amongst other factors. The disparities in cancer between the more developed and less developed countries can be seen in the etiology, late presentation and diagnosis, limited access to treatment, and limited access to opioid analgesics.

5.1.1.1. Etiology

25% of cancer deaths are caused by infectious agents.

Lecture notes by the editors:

According to the National Cancer Institute, infectious agents that can cause cancer or increase the risk of cancer include viruses, bacteria, and parasites. Some of these infectious agents cause cancer by disrupting signaling that normally keeps cell growth and proliferation in check. Other infectious agents may weaken the immune system's ability to combat cancer-causing infections. Infectious agents may also cause chronic inflammation, which may lead to cancer. Examples of infectious agents highlighted by the National Cancer Institute include the Epstein–Barr virus (EBV), hepatitis B virus and hepatitis C virus (HBV and HCV), human immunodeficiency virus (HIV), human papillomaviruses (HPVs), human T-cell leukemia/lymphoma virus type 1 (HTLV-1), Kaposi sarcoma-associated herpes virus (KSHV), Merkel cell polyomavirus (MCPyV), *Helicobacter pylori* (*H. pylori*), *Opisthorchis viverrini*, and *Schistosoma hematobium*.

Epstein–Barr virus (EBV). This is a type of herpes virus, which has been shown to cause mononucleosis (the kissing disease) as well as certain types of lymphoma and cancers of the nose and throat. The most common transmission mode for EBV is via contact with saliva e.g. through kissing, sharing toothbrushes, or cups for drinking. It is also reportedly spread by sexual contact, or blood transfusions, and organ transplantation. Unfortunately, EBV infection usually lasts a lifetime. Over 90% of the world's population is infected with EBV during their lifetime, but most do not develop any symptoms. Currently there are no treatments or vaccines for preventing EBV infection.

Hepatitis B virus and hepatitis C virus (HBV and HCV). HBV or HCV infections increase the risk of liver cancer. These viruses are transmitted via blood, e.g. via blood transfusions or when sharing needles, as well as from mother to baby during birth. HBV can also be transmitted via sexual contact. Vaccination is crucial for preventing HBV infection and is usually a requirement for healthcare workers or professionals who work in areas with human blood. There is still no vaccine against HCV. However, there are now therapies that can cure HCV infection.

Human immunodeficiency virus (HIV). The acquired immunodeficiency syndrome (AIDS) is caused by the HIV virus. HIV weakens the immune system, which may make your body more vulnerable to other infectious agents that cause cancer. However, it does not cause cancer by itself. HIV would also increase risks of a number of cancers, especially Kaposi sarcoma, lymphomas (including both non-Hodgkin lymphoma and Hodgkin disease), and cervical cancer, anal, lung, liver, prostrate, and throat cancers. HIV is transmitted via sexual contact or blood, with the highest risk being for individuals conducting unprotected sex with multiple individuals or sharing needles for injecting drugs. Currently highly effective antiviral treatment is available for those who test positive for HIV.

Human papillomaviruses (HPVs). Nearly all cervical cancers are caused by infection with high-risk types of HPV. Other cancers caused by HPVs include vaginal, vulvar, oropharyngeal, and penile cancers. High-risk HPVs are readily spread via direct sexual contact, including vaginal, oral, and anal sex. There are currently vaccines for preventing infection. In the United States, it is recommended that children be vaccinated at age 11 or 12. However, the vaccination is also suitable for individuals from ages 9 through 26. Cervical cancer screening is typically used to detect HPV infections in the cervix. While HPV infections have no treatment, the cervical abnormalities caused by these infections can be treated.

Human T-cell leukemia/lymphoma virus type 1 (HTLV-1). HTLV-1 is capable of causing T-cell leukemia/lymphoma. This virus is transmitted via blood, e.g. blood transfusions or shared needles, unprotected sex, from mother to child in the womb, or during breastfeeding. Countries where such infections are common include the Caribbean, Africa, Japan, and South America. Currently, there are no vaccines for preventing infection and no treatment is available.

Kaposi sarcoma-associated herpes virus (KSHV). This virus can cause Kaposi sarcoma, primary effusion lymphoma, and multicentric Castleman disease. The most common form of transmission is via saliva, but it can also be transmitted during organ or bone marrow transplantation and possibly through blood transfusion. KSHV is relatively common in sub-Saharan Africa, and certain regions of central and South America, where spread via saliva between family members is considered to be to be a mode of transmission. KSHV is reportedly spread by contact among children and poorly defined means amongst adults in Mediterranean countries like Greece, Israel, Saudi Arabia, and Italy. Meanwhile it can also be spread sexually by men having sex with other men in countries such as the United States and Northern Europe, where the virus is less common. Nonetheless, most people infected with this virus do not develop cancer but people with HIV infection or immunosuppression have an increased chance of developing disease. Currently there is no vaccine to prevent KSHV infection and no treatments are available. It is recommended that men who have sex with men do not conduct oral–anal contact, such as using saliva as a lubricant. Individuals with HIV could also use antiretroviral therapy to reduce risks of infection.

Merkel cell polyomavirus (MCPyV). This virus may cause a skin cancer called Merkel cell carcinoma. MCPyV affects most adults, which is most likely spread through skin-to-skin contact and indirectly by contact with contaminated or infected surfaces. There is increased risk for developing Merkel cell carcinoma for people affected by HIV or conditions suppressing the immune system. There is currently no treatment.

Helicobacter pylori (H. pylori). This is a bacterium that may cause stomach cancer called noncardia gastric cancer, or gastric MALT lymphoma. This bacterium is transmitted by consuming contaminated food or water and via mouth-to-mouth contact. According to the United States Center for Disease Control, about two-thirds of the world's population is infected by *H. pylori*. Infections are higher in LMICs. Antibiotics can be used to treat infection.

Parasitic worms. Flatworms such as *Opisthorchis viverrini* and *Schistosoma hematobium* may cause cancer of the bile ducts in the liver. These worms are often found in habitats in Southeast Asia, the Middle East, and Africa. Transmission of *Opisthorchis viverrini* is typically by eating raw meat, or poorly cooked freshwater fish containing larvae. Meanwhile, *Schistosoma hematobium* can cause bladder cancer, with transmission via free-swimming flatworm larvae burrowing into skin that has come into contact with contaminated fresh water. Antiparasitic drugs are used to treat infections by these parasitic worms.

5.1.1.2 Late presentation and diagnosis

Eighty to ninety per cent of cancer cases in LMICs are in advanced stages at diagnosis. In the case of LMICs in Africa, late presentation increases the cost of treatment and greatly reduces the chances of a cure. Factors identified as contributing to late presentation may include lack of access to healthcare, little awareness, negative symptom interpretation, fear, belief in alternative medicine, social relations and networks, amongst other compounding factors such as poor information about cancer, poor healthcare systems, limited resources, cultural and religious beliefs, illiteracy, poverty, societal priorities, lack of public education programs, and so forth.

5.1.1.3 Limited access to treatment and medicines

In sub-Saharan Africa, only 5% of cancer patients have access to chemotherapy. About half of the countries have one or no radiotherapy machine, which are used in the treatment of over 50% of cancer patients in the USA. These disparities in access to treatment have been well studied and reported on as the 'cancer divide'. Limited access to opioid analgesics is also an issue faced by LMICs in contrast to high income countries (HICs). Only 60% and 11% in middle income countries and low income countries, respectively, have access to opioid analgesics, in what is now being characterized as the pain divide.

5.1.2 Cancer prevention

Lecture notes by the editors:

> Prevention is better than cure. According to the Prevent Cancer Foundation, only five percent of cancers are hereditary. This means that the lifestyle choices we make, environmental circumstances, the foods we eat, our physical activity levels, amongst other things, directly determine our overall risk of getting cancer. Preventable cancers through lifestyle changes, or early detection and treatment include: breast, cervical, colorectal, head and neck, liver, lung, skin, testicular, and viral cancers. In general, it is believed that 30%–40% of cancers can be prevented, and one-third of cancers can be cured through early diagnosis and treatment.

The risks of developing cancers can be greatly reduced by reducing exposure to cancer risk factors: stopping tobacco use and avoiding exposure to passive smoke, minimizing alcohol consumption and exposure to the Sun, regular physical activity, eating healthily, and protecting against cancer infection agents. Screening for treatable cancers, e.g. cervical and breast cancers, could also save lives (figure 5.2).

Amongst the 'best buys' for cancer prevention are tobacco control and the HPV vaccination.

5.1.3 Tobacco strategy

5.1.3.1 Tobacco toll

Smoking is a major cause of preventable death worldwide. There are over 1.3 billion smokers worldwide, most of them in LMICs. One in two regular smokers die of smoking-related diseases, about 6 million deaths each year. Compared to non-smokers, smokers shortened their life expectancy by greater than or equal to ten years (all smokers) and about 20 years due to death from smoking-related diseases in middle age [1]. Smoking is also highly addictive with no benefit. Smoking killed 100 million people in the twentieth century, and it is expected will kill one billion people in the twenty-first century unless governments take urgent action. Smoking is a common risk factor for cancer, heart disease, and diabetes.

5.1.3.2 Tools to promote cessation and discourage initiation: MPOWER

The WHO Framework Convention on Tobacco Control (WHO FCTC) is the first global health treaty negotiated under the auspices of the World Health Organization. According to WHO, the FCTC is evidence-based, affirming that all people have the right to the highest standard of health. It is a major departure from previous approaches developing a regulatory strategy to address addictive substance, whereby the FCTC asserts the importance of demand reduction strategies as well as supply reduction issues. The framework involves 179 parties, and includes actions governments should take to address consumption of tobacco (figure 5.3).

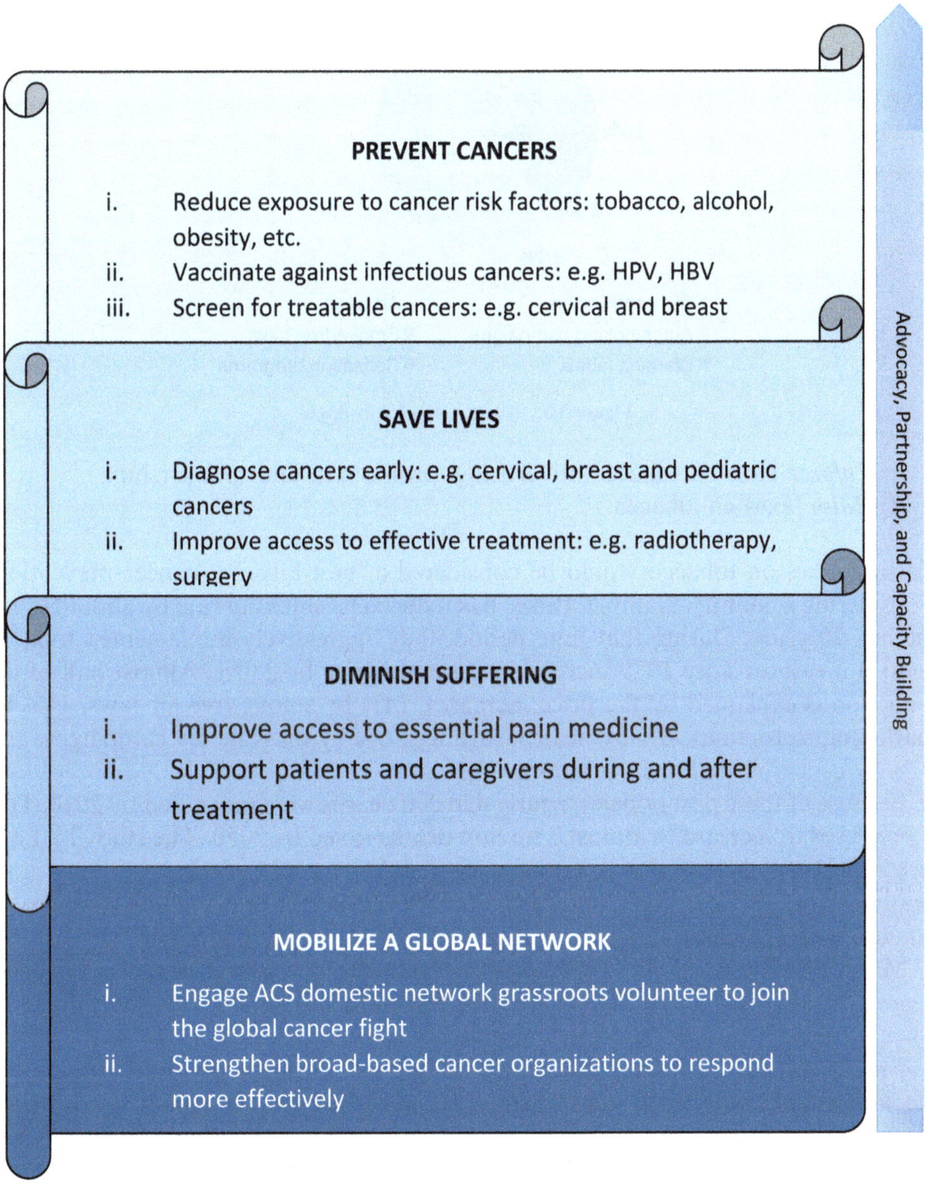

Figure 5.2. Cancer prevention illustrated.

In 2008, WHO introduced the MPOWER measures to assist in country-level implementation of the WHO FCTC provisions. MPOWER measures included:

M: *Monitor* tobacco use and prevention policies.
P: *Protect* people from tobacco smoke.
O: *Offer* help to quit tobacco use.
W: *Warn* about the dangers of tobacco.

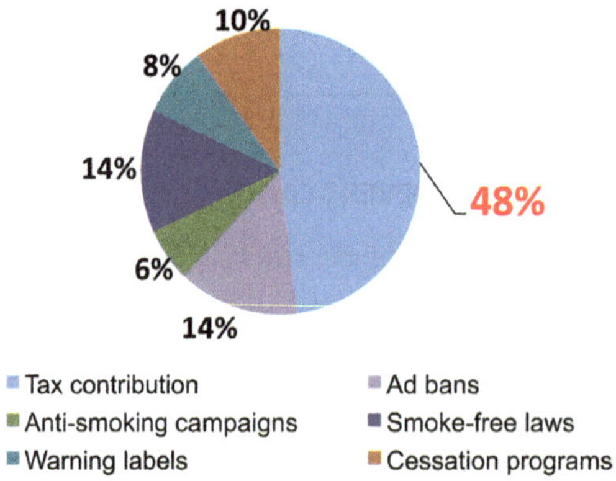

Figure 5.3. Tobacco control in Brazil.

E: *Enforce* bans on tobacco advertising, promotion, and sponsorship.
R: *Raise* taxes on tobacco.

Raising taxes on tobacco would be considered a 'best buy' for cancer prevention. Considering a country example, Brazil has reduced its smoking rate by about 50% in the last 20 years. During that time period, they aggressively implemented tobacco control measures since 1989 increasing cigarette price by 230%. Almost half of the reduction is explained by the price increases, 14% by smoke-free air laws, 14% by marketing restrictions, 8% by health warnings, 6% by mass media campaigns, and 10% by cessation treatment programs [2].

Because of these past policies, nearly 420 000 deaths were prevented by 2010. This is projected to increase to almost 7 million deaths saved by 2050. The study by Levy *et al* [2] also indicates that a set of stricter policies could prevent millions more deaths. Brazil provides an outstanding public health success story in reducing deaths due to smoking, which can be scaled or replicated in other LMICs.

Major benefits in smoking cessation have also been reported in a *New England Journal of Medicine* article. According to this study [1], smokers who quit at 25 to 34 years of age (median, 29), resulted in nearly identical life expectancy to those who had never smoked, meaning that those who quit smoking gained about ten years of life, as compared with those who continued to smoke. Survival was relatively worse for smokers who quit between 35 to 44 years of age (median, 39) than for those who had never smoked. Nonetheless, smokers who quit smoking would gain about nine years of life, as compared with those who continued to smoke. Thus, cessation at about 39 years of age reduced the excess risk of death from any cause by about 90%. Smokers who stopped smoking at 45 to 54 years of age or 55 to 64 years of age (median, 49 and 59 years, respectively) gained about six and four years of life, respectively.

5.1.4 HPV vaccination

Another 'best buy' in cancer prevention is HPV vaccination. Infections cause 16% of cancers worldwide, 2 million cases/year. Twelve high-risk oncogenic HPV types are responsible for nearly all cervical cancers (530 000 cancer cases/year), 40%–90% of vaginal, vulvar, penile, and anal cancers, and 26% of oropharyngeal cancers. HPV 16/18 infections account for 70% of cervical cancers and 90% of remaining HPV-related cancers. In comparison HPV 6/11 (low risk) cause 90% of genital warts.

Forty-five countries have introduced the HPV vaccine nationally as of 2013. The cost of vaccine (US$100 per dose) is a major barrier to the introduction of the vaccine in LMICs. In 2000 Gavi (the Vaccine Alliance) was created as an international organization to improve access to new and underused vaccines for children living in the world's poorest countries. This Vaccine Alliance brings together the public and private sectors with the common goal of creating equal access to vaccines for children, wherever they live. Gavi has made it possible for low income countries to access the HPV vaccine at a low price (US$4.50 per dose). Since 2013, GAVI has funded HPV vaccine demonstration projects in over 20 countries and funds the national HPV vaccine program in Rwanda. There is real-world evidence of the effectiveness of the HPV vaccination. Australia introduced a three-dose HPV vaccine in 2007. After the introduction of the vaccination program, a significant decrease in the incidence of high-grade cervical abnormalities was reported in girls younger than 18 years [3].

5.1.5 Advocacy

As John R Seffrin of the American Cancer Society Cancer Action Network (ACS CAN) states: 'The ultimate conquest of cancer is as much a matter of public policy as it is a medical and scientific challenge.' This statement highlights the importance of advocacy, particularly at the level of government: state legislature, congress, and country government leaders. Everyone can participate in advocacy, which is driven by research. CAN aims to:

- Fund aggressive grassroots, lobbying, and media campaigns to make every state smoke-free, to increase tobacco taxes and funding for cancer research, and advocate for early detection programs such as mammograms and colon or cervical cancer screenings.
- Supporting sophisticated training programs for volunteers to strengthen the advocacy movement and ensure that advocate voices are truly heard in the halls of government.
- Producing voter guides, candidate forums, and advertising to get every lawmaker and candidate for public office on the record in support of the things we know will fight cancer and save lives.

These model can be replicated in LMICs. ACS partners with the World Lung Foundation to produce the *Tobacco Atlas*; and the WHO and Union for International Cancer Control to produce the *Cancer Atlas*. The *Tobacco Atlas*/*Cancer Atlas* reports graphically detail the scale of the cancer and tobacco burden, progress that has been made in cancer and tobacco control, the costs of the disease, and highlights advocacy opportunities to curb the epidemic. Language editions include English, French, Arabic, Spanish, and Madarin.

The ACS CAN Mission for Global Health includes: influencing US Government policy, building a domestic grassroots network, supporting global policy change, and providing technical assistance to partners. Part of the global strategy is to support young professionals from LMICs with: leadership and advocacy training; mentorship by experienced advocates; exposure to scientific conferences and global networking opportunities; and seed grants to run advocacy campaigns.

In summary, there is a need to understand the key drivers of disparity in cancer burden between poor and rich countries, recognize the 'best buys' in prevention (taxing tobacco and the HPV vaccine) and 'best buys' in advocacy, which are evidence-based grassroots movements and youth empowerment.

5.2 Public health oncology: an ounce of prevention

Lecture by Ophira Ginsburg (World Health Organization); co-edited by Omoruyi Credit Irabor.

Cancer is a leading cause of death and disabilities worldwide, with increasing incidence and mortality cases in all income levels across the globe [4]. Factors responsible for this growth include the aging population and the adoption of lifestyle behaviors that increase cancer risk as LMICs are undergoing an economic transition, which includes industrialization, a societal shift in gender roles, as well as increased access to international markets [4]. As a result, many cancer risk factors, such as tobacco use, physical inactivity, obesity, and reproductive patterns, already prevalent in high income countries (HICs), are becoming increasingly common in LMICs [4]. Many cancers, however, can be prevented [5]. Others are detectable at an early stage in their development, and can be treated and cured. Even with late stage cancer, the pain can be reduced and the progression of the cancer slowed [6]. Cancer control is a systematic implementation of evidence-based interventions for prevention, early detection, diagnosis, treatment, and palliative management of cancers [6]. A comprehensive cancer control is one that addresses the whole population while responding to the needs of different subgroups at risk [6]. The World Health Organization (WHO) is a global voice for cancer control, playing a prominent role in the non-communicable disease (NCD) agenda because of its credibility, and field and technical expertise [7]. The WHO is the only global health body accountable to member states, and in some ways is uniquely positioned to address global cancer control via its roles in setting norms and standards (i.e. guidelines), setting research priorities, and in global health policy. The best known example of this is in the Framework Convention on Tobacco Control (FCTC), but also in influencing policies aimed at slowing the rise in obesity, physical inactivity, and alcohol use [7]. In 2013, the WHO action plan for cancer control embedded in the Global Action Plan for the Prevention and Control of NCDs 2013–2020 (resolution WHA66.10) was endorsed by the 66th World Health Assembly [8]. The Global Health Catalyst (GHC) conferences at Harvard Medical School in 2016 brought together stakeholders in the cancer control continuum and served as an avenue to learn from the experience of experts who have worked on adopting the WHO strategies for cancer control in LMICs.

5.2.1 The global cancer burden

Christiana *et al*, using the global burden of disease (GBD) methodology, estimated 17.5 million new cancer cases, 208.3 million disability life-years (DALYs), and 8.7 million deaths that were due to cancer in 2015 [9]. This statistics infers a 33% increase in cancer incidence from 2005 to 2015, of which 12.6% was due to population growth, 16.4% due to an aging population, and 4.1% due to increasing age-specific incidence rates [9]. Cancers of the respiratory system, such as tracheal, bronchus, and lung cancer, were the leading cause of cancer mortality and disability in males (1.2 million deaths and 25.9 million DALYs). Breast cancer (2.4 million cases) was the most common cancer and also the leading cause of cancer mortality and disability (523 000 deaths and 15.1 million DALYs) in females [9]. Many countries experienced a decrease in cancer mortality despite an increasing incidence rate within the ten year period. These were dominantly sub-Saharan African countries where, with a few exceptions, the healthcare infrastructure required to treat cancer is unavailable [9]. Cancer incidence is projected to further increase to 15 million in the year 2020 and 23.6 million worldwide each year by 2030, with slightly more growth in LMICs (66% more cases in 2030 than 2012) than in HICs (56% more cases in 2030 than 2012) [10]. As a result, LMICs will account for 70% of cancer cases and 33% of cancer mortality by 2030. This transition is largely attributable to the aging of populations; the adoption of modifiable risk factors for cancer (such as smoking, diet, and physical inactivity) in LMICs; and the decline in cancers related to infectious etiologies [11].

5.2.2 Risk factors for cancer

Knowledge of the causes of any particular cancer is essential in planning control. Figure 5.4 highlights the known major causes of cancers by the percentage of new cases that are attributable to each risk factor, based on data published in 1996 by the Harvard Report for Cancer Prevention [12, 13].

1. *Tobacco use.* Smoking is the single largest known contributor to cancer mortality and also the leading cause of death from the totality of major non-communicable diseases [14]. Tobacco kills approximately 6 million people and generates more than half a trillion dollars of economic damage each year [15, 16]. The WHO statistics reports 1.1 billion people, predominantly male, smoked in 2015 [16]. Although declining worldwide and in many countries, the prevalence of tobacco smoking appears to be increasing in the WHO Eastern Mediterranean Region and the African Region [13]. A country-level analysis in selected African countries estimates smoking prevalence rates of 37.7% in Sierra Leone, 34.1% in Lesotho, 28.5% in Madagascar; and less than 10% in Ethiopia, Benin, Ghana, Nigeria, and Sao Tome and Principe [17]. If this trend continues until 2020, 9 million people might die from tobacco-related causes, and over 75% of these will be in developing countries [14].
2. *Diet, body weight, and physical activity.* Diet, body weight, and activity levels promote or reduce cancer risk [14]. Cohort studies worldwide linked obesity to cancer incidence overall and to specific cancer sites that include endometrial, postmenopausal breast, colon, and esophageal adenocarcinoma [18].

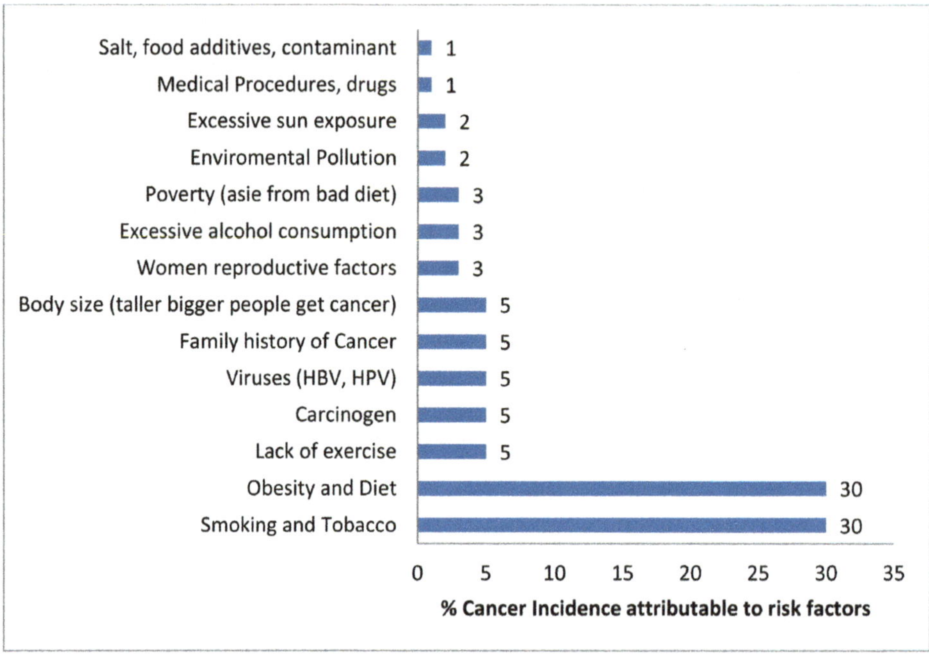

Figure 5.4. Causes of cancer. Data source [12, 13].

3. *Alcohol.* At least 183 case–control studies and 46 cohort studies have investigated alcohol's effect on the risk of developing cancer at a total of 19 sites in the body and all body sites combined [19]. Cancers of the oral cavity, larynx, liver, pharynx, breast, and esophagus, are linked to heavy alcohol use, with the risk varying by cancer site, increasing with greater intake and resulting in an estimated five percent of attributable cancer deaths in LMICs [14, 19].
4. *Infectious agents.* The three major cancer-causing infections follow tobacco in importance as risk factors for cancer incidence in developing countries. They are the human papillomavirus (HPV), hepatitis B (HBV) and hepatitis C (HCV) viruses, and *Helicobacter pylori* [14]. Oncogenic viral infections are responsible for up to 20% of cancer deaths in LMICs [20].
5. *Other causes and risk factors.* Other causes of cancers include family history, female reproductive factors, excessive Sun exposure, environmental pollution, carcinogens, and many more [14] (see figure 5.4).

5.2.3 Cancer prevention and control

The cancer control continuum (see figure 5.5) is a description of the various stages of cancer control, from cancer prevention, early detection, diagnosis, treatment, to survivorship and end-of-life care. The United Nations (UN), through WHO and its affiliates, including the International Agency for Research on Cancer (IARC) and the International Atomic Energy Agency (IAEA), support cancer control on a global

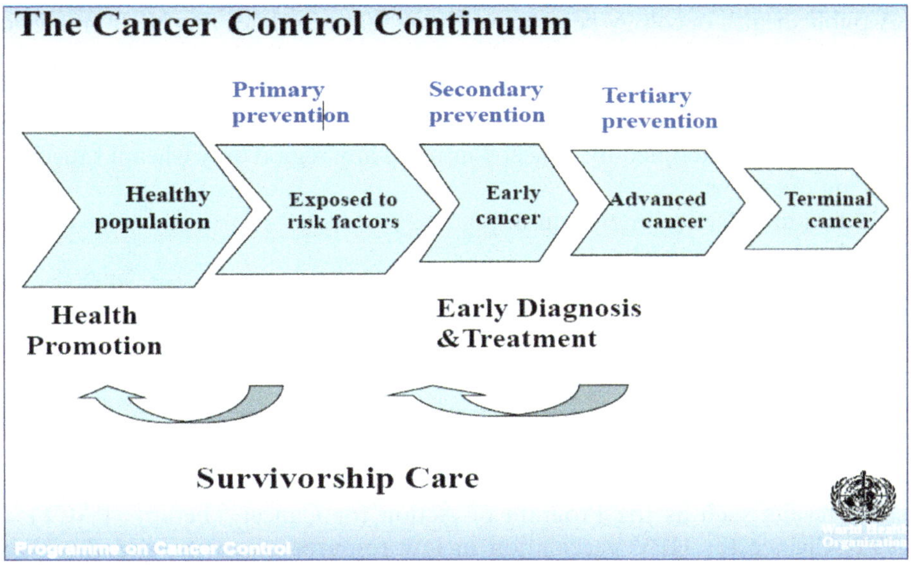

Figure 5.5. Cancer control continuum

scale [21]. The WHO sets norms and standards for control and offers technical assistance for prevention and research activities [21]. The IAEA enhances technical cooperation for radiation therapy, and the IARC developed and supports a robust cancer registry known as Globocan [21]. A number of other national and international bodies also play a significant role in raising awareness and in promoting cancer control. These include the National Cancer Institute (NCI) and its Center for Global Health, now a WHO Collaborating Center, the International Network for Cancer Treatment and Research, the National Health Institute, the International Union Against Cancer (UICC), the American Cancer Society (ACS), and other local and international cancer societies and international advocacy groups [21].

5.2.4 WHO cancer control programs

In the past few decades, WHO has developed and supported a policy framework for cancer control, known as the National Cancer Control Program (NCCP), which is currently in the 2013–2020 Global Action Plan for the prevention and control of non-communicable diseases (NCD) [8]. This new Global Action Plan and its monitoring framework were developed through consultations with the WHO Member States and stakeholders, and endorsed by the World Health Assembly in 2013 to achieve six objectives as a path to reducing the NCD burden [8]:

1. International cooperation and advocacy.
2. Country-led multi-sectorial response.
3. Risk factors and determinant.
4. Health systems and universal health coverage.
5. Research, development, and innovation.
6. Surveillance and monitoring.

A public health oncology perspective is one that translates this NCD framework into specific strategies that minimize population and individual exposure to cancer risk factors which either overlap or go beyond other NCDs. Current models for cancer control are in a series of policy menu options published in the Global Action Plan. A strategy is adopted for cancer control in any region only when it satisfies the following questions:

1. Is it an effective intervention?
2. Is it cost-effective?
3. Is it acceptable and feasible to implement?
4. Does it entail policies or individual responsibility for behavior change?
5. Can we ensure sustainability, equity?

In order to meet these needs, cancer control planners work from both the healthcare system and population-based social medicine perspectives [7]. Coordinated global partnerships are also indispensable. Collaborative efforts have yielded results such as the Program of Action for Cancer Therapy (PACT), the GAVI Alliance for HPV vaccination in low resource countries, and the United Nations Population Fund engagement in developing health systems for the early detection of cervical cancer [7].

5.2.5 Policy plan for cancer control

The policies and strategies in the Global Action Plan are for cost-effective interventions in prevention and control of NCDs in line with the set objectives. In cancer prevention, this entails both an overall preventive strategy for all cancers as well as for specific types of cancer. Policy actions in the Global Action Plan that are relevant to cancer control are highlighted in table 5.1.

5.2.6 Lessons from the field

A. Do no harm (*primum non nocere*)
   This principle holds that cancer policy planners and healthcare providers must only adopt control strategies that do no harm to the population as a whole.
B. The need for program evaluation.

Program evaluation is essential for achieving the desired results in cancer control. It improves program services and disseminates information to others regarding program successes or failures. It involves the systematic collection of information that assists public health workers to understand a program better, improve its effectiveness, and make decisions about future program planning. An evaluation can occur at different phases during the life of a program implementation:

- *Needs assessment.* An evaluation conducted before the program begins, as the first step of determining the gap in cancer control and assessing how to close the gap. For example a need assessment for national HPV vaccination.

Table 5.1. Objectives and Policy actions for global cancer control.

Objectives	Policy actions
Objective 1. (International cooperation and advocacy)	i. Raise public and political awareness, understanding and practice about prevention of cancer. ii. Integrate cancer control into the social and development agenda and poverty alleviation strategies. iii. Strengthen international cooperation for resource mobilization, capacity-building, health workforce training, and exchange of information on lessons learnt and best practices. iv. Engage and mobilize civil society and the private sector as appropriate and strengthen international cooperation to support implementation of the action plan at global, regional, and national levels. v. Implement other policy options in objective 1.
Objective 2. (Country-led multi-sectorial response)	i. Prioritize and increase, as needed, budgetary allocations for prevention and control of NCDs, without prejudice to the sovereign right of nations to determine taxation and other policies. ii. Assess national capacity for prevention and control of NCDs. iii. Develop and implement a national multi-sectorial policy and plan for the prevention and control of NCDs through multi-stakeholder engagement. iv. Implement other policy options in objective 2 paragraph 30) to strengthen national capacity including human and institutional capacity, leadership, governance, multi-sectorial action and partnerships for prevention and control of cancers.
Objective 3. (Risk factors and determinant)	TOBACCO USE i. Implement WHO FCTC. Parties to the WHO FCTC are required to implement all obligations under the treaty in full; all Member States that are not Parties are encouraged to look to the WHO FCTC as the foundational instrument in global tobacco control. ii. Reduce affordability of tobacco products by increasing tobacco excise taxes. iii. Create by law completely smoke-free environments in all indoor workplaces, public places, and public transport. iv. Warn people of the dangers of tobacco and tobacco smoke through effective health warnings and mass media campaigns. v. Ban all forms of tobacco advertising, promotion, and sponsorship. HARMFUL USE OF ALCOHOL Implement the WHO global strategy to reduce harmful use of alcohol (see objective 3, paragraphs 42, 43) through actions in the recommended target areas including: i. Strengthening awareness of alcohol-attributable cancer burden. ii. Leadership and political commitment to reduce the harmful use of alcohol. iii. Providing prevention and treatment interventions for those at risk of or affected by alcohol use disorders and associated conditions.

iv. Supporting communities in adopting effective approaches and interventions to prevent and reduce the harmful use of alcohol.
v. Implementing effective drink-driving policies and countermeasures.
vi. Regulating commercial and public availability of alcohol.
vii. Restricting or banning alcohol advertising and promotions.
viii. Using pricing policies such as excise tax increases on alcoholic beverages.
ix. Reducing the negative consequences of drinking and alcohol intoxication, including by regulating the drinking context and providing consumer information.
x. Reducing the public health impact of illicit alcohol and informally produced alcohol by implementing efficient control and enforcement systems.
xi. Developing sustainable national monitoring and surveillance systems using indicators, definitions, and data collection procedures compatible with WHO's global and regional information systems on alcohol and health.

UNHEALTHY DIET AND PHYSICAL INACTIVITY

i. Implement the WHO Global Strategy on Diet, Physical Activity and Health.
ii. Increase consumption of fruit and vegetables.
iii. Provide more convenient, safe, and health-oriented environments for physical activity.
iv. Implement recommendations on the marketing of foods and non-alcoholic beverages to children.
v. Implement the WHO global strategy for infant and young child feeding.
vi. Reduce salt intake.
vii. Replace trans fats with unsaturated fats.
viii. Implement public awareness programs on diet and physical activity.
ix. Replace saturated fat with unsaturated fat,
x. Manage food taxes and subsidies to promote healthy diet,
xi. Implement other policy options listed in objective 3 for addressing unhealthy and physical inactivity.

Objective 4. (Health systems and universal health coverage)

i. Integrate very cost-effective non-communicable disease interventions into the basic primary healthcare package with referral systems to all levels of care to advance the universal health coverage agenda.
ii. Explore viable health financing mechanisms and innovative economic tools supported by evidence.
iii. Scale up early detection and coverage, prioritizing very cost-effective high-impact interventions including cost-effective interventions to address behavioral risk factors.
iv. Train health workforce and strengthen capacity of health system particularly at the primary care level to address the prevention and control of non-communicable diseases.

(Continued)

Table 5.1. (*Continued*)

Objectives	Policy actions
	v. Improve availability of affordable basic technologies and essential medicines, including generics, required to treat major non-communicable diseases, in both public and private facilities. vi. Implement other cost-effective interventions and policy options in objective 4 to strengthen and orient health systems to address non-communicable diseases and risk factors through people-centered primary healthcare and universal health coverage. vii. Develop and implement a palliative care policy using cost-effective treatment modalities, including opioids analgesics for pain relief and training health workers. CANCER SPECIFIC STRATEGIES i. Prevention of liver cancer through hepatitis B immunization. ii. Prevention of cervical cancer through screening (visual inspection with acetic acid [VIA] or Pap smear (cervical cytology)). iii. Vaccination against human papillomavirus, as appropriate if cost-effective and affordable, according to national programs and policies. iv. Population-based cervical cancer screening linked with timely treatment. v. Population-based breast cancer and mammography screening (50–70 years) linked with timely treatment. vi. Population-based colorectal cancer screening, including through a fecal occult blood test, as appropriate, at age >50, linked with timely treatment. vii. Oral cancer screening in high-risk groups (e.g. tobacco users, betel-nut chewers) linked with timely treatment.
Objective 5. (Research, development, and innovation)	i. Develop and implement a prioritized national research agenda for non-communicable diseases. ii. Prioritize budgetary allocation for research on non-communicable disease prevention and control. iii. Strengthen human resources and institutional capacity for research. iv. Strengthen research capacity through cooperation with foreign and domestic research institutes. v. Implement other policy options in objective 5 to promote and support national capacity for high-quality research, development, and innovation.
Objective 6. (Surveillance and monitoring)	i. Develop national targets and indicators based on global monitoring framework and linked with a multi-sectorial policy and plan. ii. Strengthen human resources and institutional capacity for surveillance and monitoring and evaluation. iii. Establish and/or strengthen a comprehensive non-communicable disease surveillance system, including reliable registration of deaths by cause, cancer registration, periodic data collection on risk factors, and monitoring national response. iv. Integrate non-communicable disease surveillance and monitoring into national health information systems. v. Implement other policy options in objective 6 to monitor trends and determinants of non-communicable diseases and evaluate progress in their prevention and control.

- *Process evaluation.* An evaluation at the initial stage of the program to see if it is implemented as planned.
- *Outcome evaluation.* An evaluation conducted as the program matures to see if the set objectives are met.
- *Impact evaluation.* An evaluation carried out at the full maturation of a program to determine the effects the program had.

C. The need for local champions.
It is essential to employ local champions as an advocacy strategy and for the sustained support of other cancer control measures.
D. The need to develop an exit strategy and sustainability plan.

Exit strategies entail the fore-planning on how a cancer control program in an LMIC will be sustained after the executioner leaves the scene. There must be foresight on funding and health system integration.

5.3 Partnering with athletes

Lecture by Marc Williams (President and Founder of Williams Communications).

5.3.1 The role athletes can play in educating the public about cancer

How does sports effect our lives? Sport builds confidence, strength, and engenders social change, as well as fighting diseases and depression. It transcends language, nationality, race, and culture. Sport has the power to transform us as we reach our potential and live better lives. In the 1968 Olympics, American's John Carolos and Tommie Smith stood atop the medal podium shoeless, wearing only black dress socks on their feet. As the National Anthem began to play, they raised their fists in the Black Power salute to protest the racism and injustices in America. In 2014, NBA stars Lebron James, Carmelo Anthony, and Derrick Rose were joined by many NBA players wearing 'I can't breathe' tee shirts. It was their way of showing support of Eric Garner, who died after a confrontation with a New York Police Department officer and display the last words Garner uttered. The incident was caught on tape and sparked national outrage in the USA.

We also recall when other forms of images in sports captured our attention and left an indelible mark forever. Clutch performances from the likes of Michael Jordan for the University of North Carolina winning the 1982 championship. The following year in Albuquerque, on 4 April 1983, North Carolina State played against a Houston team that had been ranked No. 1 in the nation and was led by future Hall of Famers Hakeem Olajuwon and Clyde Drexler. Unknown Lorenzo Charles's game-winning shot become emblematic of the NCAA tournament and has been shown thousands of times. However, it was the image of the victorious N.C. State coach Jim Valvano, darting across the court looking for someone to hug. That moment will always be embedded in our hearts. Ten years later, on 3 March 1993, Valvano was honored with the inaugural Arthur Ashe Courage and Humanitarian Award at the ESPY Awards after a stellar coaching and broadcaster career. Valvano had been diagnosed with metastatic adenocarcinoma metastatic a year earlier and died weeks after delivering his impassionate speech at the ESPY Awards and the power of that speech still lives on [22]:

> 'Cancer can take away all of my physical abilities. It cannot touch my mind, it cannot touch my heart, and it cannot touch my soul. And those three things are going to carry on forever [23].'

Jim Valvano's message shared a common connection with cancer patients, spurred by the warrior mentality any patient needs to get through treatment. His words go deeper than that, especially at a time when our country seems so divided by many issues. One of the ways many cope with daily challenges is to turn our attention to sports. Watching sports offers an escape from the daily grind of work and life. Sports is the arena where we root for athletes and teams, providing a sense of belonging for fans. Some would argue that cheering for a team can create a sense of pride and raise one's self-esteem. When we find out one of our sports heroes is injured or suffers a personal loss, we empathize with them and want to do more to support them—in some cases more than we want to do for our own loved ones—that is the power sport has in our society.

What I remembered the most that evening about that speech was Valvano's alarming numbers about cancer: 'The Arthur Ashe Foundation is a wonderful thing and the amount pouring in for AIDS is not enough but it is TEN times the amount that goes into cancer research. One in every four will be afflicted by this disease. We (ESPN) are starting the Jimmy V Foundation for Cancer Research and the motto is "Don't give up…Don't ever give up!"' [22].

The number has narrowed 15 years later according to Dr Will Ngwa, a world renowned cancer researcher from Harvard University, who says 'One in every three people has cancer or will be afflicted with it.' This is an alarming statistic, and many of us have family and friends with this deadly disease. Many of them suffer in silence along with countless millions victimized globally. In our daily lives we tend to want to escape and have a distraction from all the chaos we are faced with daily. How can athletes lend support in fighting cancer?

5.3.2 Athletes' role

Today, many athletes use their voice to raise awareness about many causes, mostly about education, such as Lebron James providing over 1500 students from Akron with challenging backgrounds like his the chance to go to college for free. Other athletes such as Eli Manning and Tiger Woods have given away millions to young people to improve their lives. Coaches such as Bob Huggins of West Virginia and Jim Larranaga of the University of Miami speaking candidly about cancer. However Dikembe Mutombo is arguably the most generous athlete the world has ever seen. Aside from spending $15 million on a hospital [24] in his native Congo, he has also been recognized as a Global Ambassador for the Special Olympics. The list of charities he supports include his own Dikembe Mutombo Foundation, FACE Africa, HOPE Worldwide, Make-A-Wish Foundation, Unicef, ONE Campaign, and Right to Play. Legendary icons such as NBA Top 50 Players and Basketball Hall of Famer Rick Barry value the importance of taking care of yourself and for athletes to use their voice to educate people about diseases such as cancer, e.g. in the words of Barry:

> 'The most important gift from God we have in life is our health. I feel it is essential that we take care of ourselves, not just for us, but for our families. I have dedicated my life to achieving the most optimum health and I encourage everyone I come in contact with to do the same [24].'

Barry goes on to say,

> 'Athletes should use their celebrity platform to promote good health globally because of the impact they can have on people. Fans will listen to someone they look up to and respect. Also, more companies and brands will provide resources to help find cures for debilitating diseases [24].'

Former Superbowl Champion from the Indianapolis Colts, Marlin Jackson, says,

> 'We must place significance and value on what God has provided—our Health! What you put in, or let in, determines what you'll get out. Whether it be your mind, what you watch, what you read, or the people you surround yourself with. The same reasoning should be applied to our bodies, we've only been given one, so it's our responsibility to consciously choose wisely when making decisions pertaining to our body. What we eat determines how we feel and heel. As an athlete, I've learned the importance of placing value and priority on my health! [24]'

Eating a healthy, balanced diet can help you keep a healthy body weight. Keeping a healthy weight is important, because obesity is the second biggest preventable cause of cancer after smoking. Diet can also directly affect cancer risk. Eating healthily still does not guarantee you will not get cancer; popular ESPN Sports Anchor Stuart Scott passed away from Cancer in 2014 and was well known for having a healthy diet. It prompted his colleague and fellow sports anchor Jay Crawford to say, 'Cancer is a killer that knows no boundaries. Young. Old. Black. White. Rich. Poor. It takes all kinds. It takes all of us, TOGETHER, to fight back.'

Athletes from various sports have expressed their concern about the importance of global health and being educated about cancer. Three-time Olympian in track and field Hazel Clark says, 'The battle against cancer is very similar to what it takes to be an elite athlete; determination, faith, and resilience. Those who battle cancer are champions in the truest sense. As athletes we recognize and celebrate their strength.' Former 400 meter world-record holder and Olympic Gold Medalist Harry 'Butch' Reynolds knows what it means to have determination, faith, and resilience, as he served as a care giver to his father-in-law for eight years (who suffered from multi-myeloma) and his brother who suffered from neurosarcoidosis. 'Cancer is serious and one must have a strong mind, body and soul as well as a great support network to endure it,' says Reynolds. 'Athletes can do more by lending their voices to bring awareness and hopefully this can be the impetus to finding a cure to this disease.' Four time-Olympian, Bronze Medalist, and American Record holder in the 800 meters Johnny Gray says, 'It is imperative athletes use their amazing platform to educate and empower others to learn about deadly diseases such as cancer, we all know someone in our lives that has been affected by it. Cancer has destroyed many family members young and old, it must be stopped!'

Although it is imperative that we encourage athletes to speak out against cancer, it is also important that all people are knowledgeable about cancer. Dr Richard Southall, one of the leading sports management educators in the world, does a lot to educate people about how cancer has affected his life:

> 'My family, like so many, has been hurt by cancer. My mom, Gladys, and my brother-in-law, Steve, both died from cancer. My wife, Deb, is a uterus cancer survivor. Part of living is battling and never giving up. We all have battles in our lives. We are always stronger together.'

In addition to athletes and members of our society, it is very important that we identify organizations that raise money to find a cure for cancer. There are many sports foundations that seek to raise money for cancer but there is more work to be done.

5.3.3 Foundations in sports that fight cancer

The V Foundation has been the leading sports organization that raises money for Cancer awareness. ESPN Radio has raised more than $6.5 million to fund cancer research since the first annual Don't Give Up ESPYS V Foundation Auction in 2005, including $781 258 in 2016. ESPN's 2016 Jimmy V Week for Cancer Research celebrated its tenth year and set a new record, raising more than $3.8 million for the V Foundation for Cancer Research. Over the past ten years, Jimmy V Week fundraising totals over $17.6 million for cancer research.

As a result of the awareness ESPN's programming has brought the V Foundation for sponsors and sport fans, the Goldberg Family, BRCA Foundation, and Basser Initiative at the Gray Foundation were inspired to make a $3 million challenge during the Jimmy V Men's Classic, which aims to be matched by the V Foundation in 2017. In addition, over $300 000 was raised for the John Saunders Grant for Pediatric Cancer Research including a $100 000 grant from ESPN. The John Saunders grant was established in memory of the late ESPN anchor and founding V Foundation board member, John Saunders, who suddenly passed away in August of 2016.

Basketball iconic television personality Vitale has raised over $15 million over the past 11 years at his annual Vitale Gala and last year his team raised $2.38 million for pediatric cancer research. Each year he honors a famous coach who epitomizes the values of Jimmy Valvano.

5.3.4 Organizations for women

One of the leading organizations that fights cancer for women is The Kay Yow Cancer Fund, founded 2007 after North Carolina State University's legendary basketball coach Kay Yow. The foundation has to date raised over $6 million. Before her death, Yow joined forces with the Women's Basketball Coaches Association (WBCA) and The V Foundation for Cancer Research to form the Kay Yow Cancer Fund, committed to being a part of finding an answer in the fight against women's cancers through raising money for scientific research, assisting the underserved, and unifying people for a common cause. Brenda Nichols, Head Women's Basketball Coach at Sam Houston State who was a dear friend of Coach Yow says, 'Having been involved in sports my whole life, I believe in the power teamwork provides when battling any opponent. I personally know individuals who have fought cancer valiantly and can only imagine how supported they must feel knowing they have teams of supporters working tirelessly to bring victory against this deadly foe.'

I am reminded of Jim Valvano's plea to the 2000 plus members of the audience on 3 March 1993 at the ESPYs: 'Don't give up. Don't ever give up.' I challenge fans to encourage athletes to use their enormous platform to bring awareness to social issues, but most of all dreadful diseases and helping to find a cure for cancer. Despite his failing health, Valvano spoke for more than ten minutes about his life and his illness with a positivity and perspective that continues to inspire 20 years later [22]:

> 'I just got one last thing, I urge all of you, all of you, to enjoy your life, the precious moments you have,' Valvano said. 'To spend each day with some laughter and some thought, to get your emotions going. To be enthusiastic every day and as Ralph Waldo Emerson said, "Nothing great could be accomplished without enthusiasm [24]."'

Imagine if athletes were enthusiastic and passionate about fighting cancer and created awareness among us all. We could be much closer to a cure than you think.

Video by athletes united against cancer: www.globalhealthcatalystevents.org/multimedia.

5.4 Partnering with the resource-laden diaspora

5.4.1 The role of Africans in diaspora in sustainable health outcomes for Africa

By Terence Ngwa, Valentine Nebangwa, and Eric Tanifum.

5.4.1.1 Background

Africans in diaspora (AiD) are increasingly being recognized as a valuable resource in development efforts on the African continent. While remittances have been prominently referenced, there are development areas where diaspora involvement supports community, national, and even continent-wide development. One such area is that of healthcare. There has never been the level of urgency in addressing the health crisis in Africa as there is today. Diseases of all sorts have ravaged inhabitants of the continent at a rate that is unprecedented, with non-communicable diseases specifically being a main cause of death. While examples of diaspora contributions in the area of health development in Africa can be found, efforts of AiD to address the health needs of the continent have hitherto been fragmented, sporadic, uncoordinated, and unsustainable.

5.4.1.2 Global Health Catalyst summit: a platform for diaspora engagement

In 2015 a visionary group of healthcare, research, and philanthropy professionals led by members of the African diaspora initiated the Global Health Catalyst (GHC) summit at Harvard. This annual summit uniquely brings together experts in healthcare, research, low cost technologies, policy, and philanthropy. Among the strengths of this summit are its commitment to the education and engagement of AiD.

The 2016 GHC summit was characterized by a call to action for all Africans living in the diaspora to form a common front that would undercut the damaging effects of non-communicable diseases on the continent. During the AiD United Against Cancer breakout session on day two of the summit, a group of AiD leaders engaged in dialogue and tasked a steering group with exploring options through which the African diaspora can establish a coordinated front to lead the fight against cancer and other diseases on the African continent. During the session and a follow-up conference call a month later, members adopted the following as primary areas in which AiD can and should work towards advancement in the health sector for Africa and Africans:

- Cancer education and awareness.
- Advocacy.
- Participation in telemedicine.
- Organization of health workshops.
- Mobile clinics.
- Crowdfunding research.
- Online learning.

These avenues were chosen for their potential to generate an immediate and sustainable impact on the health needs of the African continent. More importantly, the committee members recognized that for these efforts to be effective and sustainable the AiD must leverage opportunities and its capabilities in leadership, collaborations, and diversity.

5.4.1.3 Leadership

Despite the growing participation of diaspora members in African health matters, there is a limited number of diaspora leaders to guide their efforts. The example set by leading participants at the 2016 GHC summit served as a reminder and a challenge to the AiD that they possess the skills and have a responsibility to lead efforts to reduce the health disparities that are customary on the African continent. A member of the AiD United Session shared the example of the African Affairs Advisory Group (AAAG), chaired by a Tanzanian diaspora, which serves as a liaison between African communities in Montgomery County and the county government. Through this, the

AAAG ensures that the latter effectively responds to the needs and concerns of the African immigrants living and/or working in Montgomery County. The AAAG, through its healthcare committee, has been instrumental in partnering with diaspora entities and mobilizing communities in response to the needs of the many health disparities on the continent. As a result of this effort, there was a robust response to the 2015 Ebola outbreak in West Africa through fundraising, mobilization of healthcare personnel, collection of medical supplies, outreach to educate families and friends on the ground, and a concerted effort to facilitate and support the work of non-governmental organizations operating in the region.

It is imperative that AiD spearhead these initiatives. Most, if not all Africans living in the diaspora have experienced the pain of having a family member succumb to the agony of the disease due to substandard treatment conditions. The diaspora's influence on the daily lives of their communities of origin can be extremely effective. It is within this backdrop that the fight for better health for Africa must be the diaspora's business. It is gratifying to note that some health professionals of African origin in Montgomery county Maryland as well as other counties across the US are living up to the challenge and are shining examples worth emulating. Some of them are now regulars at the GHC summit. While the number of AiD involved in African healthcare development is growing, there is a need for more leaders to emerge to direct diaspora efforts in healthcare.

5.4.1.4 Collaboration

Collaboration is one of the pillars of the GHC summit. During each summit, and in the months between summits, collaborations are forged and strengthened between participating organizations, institutions, and businesses. The AiD recognized the need for their active participation in such collaborations. A recent collaboration between the AAAG and the Patch Foundation, that will benefit both Africans living in the continent and those in the diaspora through better education on early cancer detection and treatment options, was highlighted during the AiD session. Fountain of Hope Mission and the African Renaissance Ambassador Corp are also teaming up to further cancer education, health, and wellness in Cameroon. Multiple opportunities exist for collaborations between diaspora groups, organizations, and businesses. AiD United Against Cancer strongly encourages these partnerships and collaborations, and urges other groups to follow suit. Groups that run annual health clinics in Africa are valuable assets in establishing sustainable partnerships that could be critical to positive achievements in health initiatives. Greater collaboration between the diaspora and local health practitioners were seen as having the potential to yield better results. The diaspora has tremendous potential to leverage funding from multinational companies operating in Africa and to harness the expertise and organizational know-how of existing diaspora nonprofit groups. For this reason funding proposals exhibiting collaborative approaches highlighting these diverse abilities are advisable.

5.4.1.5 Diversity

The participants of the AiD breakout session were diverse not only in terms of their African origins, but also in their professional experience and the types of development projects they are involved in. Rather than being a hindrance, this diversity made discussions livelier with interesting perspectives, examples from experience, and suggestions for alternative approaches to the common healthcare challenges that span the entire African continent. This led to the conclusion that the diversity found within the AiD community should be seen as a strength to be identified and incorporated in global health efforts. Judging from the success of the 2016 GHC summit, which brought together a wide range of presenters and participants, the AiD were encouraged to explore ways to diversify their approaches by utilizing the multiple experiences and skills of their fellow AiD. Furthermore, it was seen as imperative that the AiD take full advantage of its rich diversity and talent pool in the areas of research and development, and clinical translation, to champion the development of low-cost treatment options for cancer and diseases endemic to the continent.

5.4.1.6 Considerations for diaspora engagement

Multiple opportunities exist, such as employing social media and utilizing innovative software technologies and applications to enhance outreach to local communities. Planning education and awareness events involving social groups and schools when vacationing in Africa is another promising opportunity. Funding agencies for partnerships in healthcare and development, such as the Ford, the Bill and Melinda Gates, and the Clinton Foundations, can be explored to finance such efforts. However, the sustainability of these partnerships will rely heavily on the commitment of all partners to the projects and regular communication of results, successes, and any challenges faced in the field.

5.4.1.7 Conclusion

The AiD session at the 2016 GHC proved to be an illuminating session for all participants. The importance of the AiD taking a leadership role in global health issues is clear, particularly as concerns healthcare in Africa. Collaborative efforts within and outside the diaspora community were encouraged. Diversity was identified as a valuable tool in bringing together multiple stakeholders for far-reaching, sustainable contributions to health outcomes in Africa. Overall the AiD Session at the 2016 GHC summit served as a platform for the education and engagement of the AiD in global health efforts.

Acknowledgement

We appreciate the contributions of all AiD United Against Cancer Session Participants for their input:

Eric Tanifum, Terence Ngwa, Valentine Nebangwa, Masipula Sithole, Jackie Jua, Adejoke Sheyin, Eric Atanga, Ellis Morfaw, Jacci Kameri, Ledet Muleta, Emmanuel Chebe, Innocent Chia, Albert Agboretang, Ivan Ndamukong, Nixon Nebane, Conelius Ngwa, Harriet Shangarai, Melvin Foote, Stella-Maris Adamu, Nicoline Ambe, and Kenneth Ngwa.

5.4.2 Africans in diaspora as partners in global health: examples from the Global Health Catalyst summit

By Lydia Asana (CEO, African Renaissance Ambassador Corp).

5.4.2.1 Introduction

One thing that makes the Global Health Catalyst (GHC) summit at Harvard unique is the diversity of presentations, perspectives, and participants present at each summit. These individual puzzle pieces, as they may initially appear to be, are given a common platform through which to explore and address the growing burden that cancer and other non-communicable diseases are placing, not only on affected Africans on the continent, but also on governments, health systems, organizations, and institutions on the African continent and beyond. Development agencies all over the world are also adversely affected by the growing health disparities that exist between LMICs and the rest of the world.

While representatives of multiple groups attend the annual GHC summit, purposeful engagement of AiD has a vital significance that may be lost to healthcare, research, education, policy, philanthropy, and IT professionals with a vested interest in African development. In fact, it may be that even members of the AiD community are at a loss as to the vital role they can play in securing sustainable gains in global health for the African continent. The following is an attempt to use AiD participation at the GHC summit to illustrate the benefits that can result from active engagement of the AiD in global health efforts.

5.4.2.2 Scholarly interest in the diaspora

The contemporary African diaspora is increasingly being credited with the potential to make significant contributions to their sending nations, as a result of their ability to harmonize relationships in their sending countries with those in their countries of residence using their transnational skills and knowledge [25]. Because of this they should be included as key players in the development of the African continent. Although such sentiments have been expressed by world leaders, multilateral agencies, and social activists, questions regarding how this potential may be realized in specific areas, such as healthcare, remain. At a time when innovative solutions are sought for widespread global health concerns including cancer, diaspora populations with inherent multicultural characteristics and transnational skills may hold the key to success. While the significance and role of financial remittances by diaspora are often referenced [26], the focus on social remittances is also gaining recognition [27]. Scholars have also found that not only are AiD interested in the development of Africa, they also have a tendency to get involved in such initiatives [28].

Using examples drawn from AiD involvement with the GHC summit, this paper illustrates that the AiD are valuable in multiple ways to a number of global health stakeholders. They serve one another within AiD communities; they give back to their sending communities; they provide services to African communities outside their sending communities; they build the capacity of interested individuals worldwide; and they serve as a bridge for development to African organizations and institutions, as well as to organizations and institutions based in the United States and other parts of the world.

5.4.2.3 The GHC summit and AiD

In just two years, GHC summit participants have listed over 21 African countries as countries with which they have established professional or personal relationships. These countries include: Botswana, Burundi, Cameroon, Central African Republic, Egypt, Ethiopia, Gabon, Ghana, Kenya, Liberia, Malawi, Morocco, Nigeria, Rwanda, Senegal, Sierra Leone, South Africa, Swaziland, Sudan, Tanzania, Zambia, and Ivory Coast. Judging from such participation, the potential for this initiative to have impact across the African continent is evident. The skills, interests, and professions of summit participants as seen in the range of presentation and discussion topics at these summits provide fertile soil for collaboration. AiD leaders who attend GHC summits represent diaspora groups and organizations working in a number of fields including advocacy, cancer (screening, education, research, treatment), career development, community development, diabetes, faith and spirituality, health education, higher education, information and communication technologies (ICTs), journalism, radiation oncology, mental health, research, youth development, small business, sports, and much more. The sheer diversity of participants and topics is as good a reason as any for the AiD to attend this annual event. But what is even more important to understand about the participation of the AiD at the GHC is the valuable resource the AiD can be for Africa, for non-Africans interested in the development of Africa, and for other members of the AiD community.

5.4.2.4 AiD contributions to AiD communities

New immigrants tend to settle in areas where there is an existing community of the diaspora with whom they can identify. As such, diaspora leaders are often influential in both meeting the needs of diaspora, and making the needs of the diaspora community known to local leaders and service providers. This is something that the Montgomery County African Affairs Advisory Group is doing in Maryland. The chair of this group has been an active part of the annual GHC summits. This dynamic woman's commitment to improving health outcomes for African populations is seen in her Nesi Wangu health blog, which provides life-saving health information to Africans at home and abroad in the Swahili language.

AiD leaders are able to relate to others in the diaspora community and gain their trust in a way that others may not be able to. This advantage can be utilized in particularly sensitive areas such as mental health, where cultural influences often interfere with the pursuit of medical attention. The 2016 GHC summit provided a platform for the founder of Barak Village to present her mental health initiative sharing about a service that many diaspora communities fail to seek. Medixaa an organization that uses media to promote mental health awareness, and Rhythm for Recovery, which seeks to employ the arts in mental health treatment, were also present illustrating the AiD's interest and ability to venture into hitherto taboo areas of global health.

The AiD United Against Cancer Breakout Session at the 2016 GHC summit gathered AiD leaders for a targeted discussion to identify key areas where diasporans can play an active part in efforts to advance cancer care, education, and research in Africa. Through contributions to this discussion, AiD leaders served as a resource to one another and further explored ways in which their diverse backgrounds and areas of work can be channeled into complimentary, collaborative global health efforts. Examples of the diverse sectors present included business (HopeLand Group), public policy (Constituency for Africa), higher education (Association of Nigerian Women Academic Doctors Inc.), women's associations (African Women's Cancer Awareness Association), journalism (Dunia Magazine), as well AiD working in the fields of scientific research, healthcare, writing, accounting, management, education, and nonprofit management.

5.4.2.5 AiD support their sending countries

Literature documenting the efforts of diaspora associations often highlights the support system this provides for diasporans as well as the development projects they initiate in their sending countries. The Diaspora Council of Tanzanians in America (DICOTA) was presented at the 2016 GHC summit as one such organization. In addition to members of the Tanzania diaspora serving as a resource within their diaspora and to their sending nation, the Tanzania diaspora was presented as a pool of human resources that can be tapped for development projects in a number of fields including health, something the former Tanzania Ambassador to the US must have recognized as she presented a keynote address at the 2015 GHC summit. Professional societies such as the Ethio-American Doctors Group provide sector-specific expertise, support, and vision that bring resources, infrastructure, and services to their sending nations. At the 2015 GHC summit, a presentation by a representative of this association of medical personnel hailing from Ethiopia showed how effective such associations can be. Their project to construct a state-of-the-art hospital in Ethiopia, is moving from vision to reality.

5.4.2.6 AiD support African nations

AiD tend to support not only their sending communities, but also have a tendency to support development on the African continent in general. One of the organizations through which this is done, the Patcha Foundation, shared information on their annual medical missions to African nations with participants of both the 2015 and 2016 GHC summits. Their mission teams regularly include African diaspora healthcare professionals who give of their time and talents to serve anywhere a medical mission is planned.

5.4.2.7 AiD build capacity worldwide

The African Organizations for Research and Training in Cancer (AORTIC) has been involved in both the 2015 and 2016 GHC summits. During the 2016 summit AORTIC launched its online educational platform, which will increase the number of individuals who benefit from the instruction of seasoned AORTIC professionals. This includes AORTIC members and other interested parties all over the world. In addition, a number of AiD leaders associated with the GHC are highly sought after educators and speakers who have presented to international audiences and multiple conferences.

5.4.2.8 AiD inform and inspire

Some of the most eye-opening and moving stories and experiences shared during GHC summits come from AiD who have experienced life in both Africa and in Western nations. The passion of these individuals runs deep as a result of personal experiences, such as their own battle with cancer, the pain of losing a loved one in Africa to a health condition that could have been treated elsewhere in the world, and stories of triumph from humble beginnings to international leadership roles. In sharing their experiences speakers, such as the founder of Cancer Africa, humanize some of the seemingly abstract challenges presented in the form of medical terms and research figures, and inspire participants in their efforts to narrow the great divide that distinguishes healthcare in LMICs from healthcare in other parts of the world.

5.4.2.9 AiD serve as a bridge to development

The transnational traits of AiD characterized by simultaneous interactions in their sending countries and in their countries of residence provide the AiD with a unique ability to identify needs on the African continent, seek resources in their countries of residence, and serve as a bridge that brings resources to needs. Diaspora members of the GHC summit exhibit this as they bring human and other resources together to address identified health needs plaguing LMICs, particularly those in Africa. Members of Medical Physicists in Diaspora (MEPHIDA) illustrated this profoundly by proactively engaging stakeholders in Cameroon with diaspora medical doctors and medical physicists, in collaboration with key members of the GHC, to further develop a roadmap for the creation of a comprehensive cancer treatment center in Cameroon.

5.4.2.10 Positive outcomes for AiD participants of the GHC summit

While much of the preceding information has focused on the value of AiD as a resource, the GHC is painfully aware that the AiD have sometimes been placated in hopes of benefitting from their development potential with little regard to providing outcomes of value to this population. While the GHC encourages groups and institutions in Africa, within AiD Communities, and of non-African origin to view the AiD as a valuable resource, the GHC summit seeks to provide a mutually beneficial experience for the AiD and the communities and organizations they represent. By providing education and information from world-renowned speakers, providing opportunities for AiD to present their projects, and facilitating networking opportunities, the GHC has also served as a resource supporting the AiD in growing their organizations and strengthening their impact. A number of positive outcomes have already been identified. Collaborative partnerships have been forged for joint projects between the GHC and a number of diaspora-led organizations and institutions, including the African Renaissance Ambassador Corp, AORTIC,

Constituency for Africa, ICT University, MEPHIDA, NesiWangu—My Nurse, and the Patcha Foundation, to name but a few.

A number of diaspora leaders who attended the 2015 GHC summit and learned about AORTIC attended the AORTIC conference in Morocco later that year, benefitting from information, training, and additional networking opportunities.

Participating groups and organizations such as the African Renaissance Ambassador Corp, NesiWangu—My Nurse, and the Patcha Foundation have also recorded gains as seen in programing and activities that reflect GHC summit themes. Mental health, addressing global gaps in cancer, and the role of ICTs in global health are three such growing areas of interest. GHC organizers are also pleased to note that speakers and other resources introduced at the GHC summit are being explored and utilized by these and other diaspora groups. By extending the knowledge and networks initiated and strengthened at GHC summits, the overarching aims of the summit, including diaspora engagement in global health, are being met and expanded.

While gains amongst diaspora groups are commendable, strides in healthcare initiatives on the African continent are also celebrated. For example, a partnership between MEPHIDA, Bingo Baptist Hospital, members of the GHC, and other stakeholders has paved the way for a roadmap to move towards plans for construction of a cancer treatment facility in Cameroon. A similar project has also been initiated with partners in Kenya. Education and awareness regarding the need for improved and increased availability of palliative care on the Africa continent is also bearing fruit, as seen by increased interest in this subject leading to expanded opportunities for palliative care sessions at future GHC summits and other events.

While these are but a few of the concrete outcomes growing out of the GHC summits, they illustrate both the value AiD bring to global health initiatives, and the resources they gain for their organizations, the diaspora, and the African populations they serve.

5.4.2.11 Conclusion

AiD have been noted for their potential to support development efforts on the African continent. Studies and examples of diaspora remittances, be they financial or social, often refer to individual efforts, hometown/country associations, and sometimes professional associations. In just two years GHC summits have illustrated the promise and possibilities that exist for AiD to make their contributions to global health, particularly global cancer efforts, as a diverse, yet united diaspora. Individual diaspora leaders, as well as diaspora-led associations, businesses, institutions, groups, and organizations, can serve as a valuable resource to the global health community while gaining resources for their specific development efforts. By serving as a platform for knowledge sharing, providing networking opportunities, and catalyzing collaborations, GHC summits have brought together the seemingly unrelated puzzle pieces of diverse people, ideas, and projects, including AiD in a way that results in mutually beneficial coordinated efforts that are shaping positive, sustainable, life-saving global health outcomes.

5.5 Partnering with religious institutions

By Kenneth Ngwa (Professor of Theology, Director of Center for Christianities in Global Contexts, Drew University).

5.5.1 Introduction: setting the health–religion table

When I picked up Colin Norman's book, *The God That Limps*, I was excited and expecting to find some discussion about religion; specifically about religion and health. That was before I had the chance to read the subtitle and discover that it was a book about technological development and its relation to shifting social identity in the global landscape, post-World War II [29]. In fairness, the main title was not completely misleading. Norman began his first chapter with some reflection on Hephaestus, the ancient Greek god of fire and metalworking, charged with keeping the ancient society running smoothly. Depicted as infirm in his legs, Hephaestus 'was the only imperfect member of the pantheon of classical gods.' Norman drew from this ironic depiction of the ancient deity to explore paradoxical attitudes towards modern forms of the ancient deity's craft, technology: technological development represented the promise of major breakthroughs that could solve (or at least mitigate) the world's enormous challenges, on the one hand. And on the other, technological development was potentially responsible for some of the ills of the world, from pollution to nuclear war [29, pp 15,16].

My initial disappointment with the subject matter (not the content) of Norman's book, however, soon turned to intrigue as I stalled just a little while to ponder the depiction of the deity. The use to Hephaestus as a gateway to Norman's reflections on technology and the metaphor of the limping deity tasked with keeping the society functioning smoothly intrigued me. The metaphor signaled an obvious truth: disability does not foreclose ability or predict inability [30], certainly not for a community that had chosen to engage and embrace its limping deity. Echoes of the legend of Sundiata of ancient Mali, crippled and exiled only to return to restore the greatness of ancient Mali (overcoming a deadly mysterious enemy, Sumanguru), comes to mind [31]. For the purposes of this essay, the metaphor of the limping deity also intrigued me in another way: how is it that the majority world, the global south, has both a high demographic of religious persons and persons without sufficient healthcare? How might attitudes about health and wellness shift if health and healthcare are intimately intertwined with religion, as co-constitutive of human wellbeing? What might a community's reaction be to healthcare needs if such needs are linked to, and understood as, part of something sacred and bigger than physical and mental infirmity? What if the sick person is not just a sick individual but rather a sick *member of a family or church or community*? What if illness and health are perceived not just as biological and mental conditions but also as social and cultural conditions?

As I reflected further, I began to think of biblical passages. Some texts (Deuteronomy 28) suggest that health, broadly understood, is a function of communal relations and bonds, and violations of those social bonds lead to physical illness and social disease. Without suggesting a professionalized medical system, biblical texts mention a variety of treatments, including bandages (Ezekiel 30:21), prayers, and mandrakes used to address infertility (Genesis 30:14). The prophet Jeremiah repeatedly speaks of the need for his community—desperately seeking healing—to get balsam from Gilead (Jeremiah 8:22; 46:11; 51:8). The writer of the epistle of James instructs the community to be engaged in facilitating healing for its sick members (James 5:14–16). Other passages raise important questions about religion and health. When the biblical text (1 Samuel 16:23) speaks of David's music functioning as a soothing mechanism for a schizophrenic Saul, is there medical validity to the claim beyond the narrative depiction of Saul's physical response to the music: his experience of health (or 'good')? When Jesus rubs mud on the eyes of a blind man and asks him to go wash and be restored (John 9:6–7), is there any physiological mechanism behind the miracle of restoration through re-engagement with the elements of his geographical and religious habitat? And what about diet? When we read in the book of Daniel that *religious dieting* has measurable physical outcomes, what exactly is the relation between the religious belief and the food (Daniel 1:2–15)? If a non-Hebrew had eaten the same food over the same period of time, would they have the same physical outcomes? The exilic prophet, Second Isaiah, depicts her anguished community gathering around the physically tortured and deformed body of one of its members, and claiming some kind of vicarious healing and new identity from their relation to the diseased body (Isaiah 53:5). One could multiply such biblical examples, but I think the point is made: there has been, since ancient times, a profound relation between religion and health, and that relation needs to be theorized anew and deployed for the healing of peoples and nations. Again and again, these texts suggest that religious communities define their identity and purpose *not simply by their response to sickness and disease, but more importantly by their relation to unwell members of the community*. Healing is deeply rooted in environmental setting, in culture and practice, in healer–patient relations, and in the symbols and rituals of religious practice. As Mary Douglas, the anthropologist and ritual theorist argued, biblical notions of holiness, wholeness, purity, dietary concerns, and bodily disease are all intertwined [32].

This brings me back to Norman's book: *The God that Limps* is an exploration of the power of symbolism and material utility in the fields of religion and technological development; it is an invitation to engage in interdisciplinary reflection, which I intend to explore in terms of religion and health. That is the space I occupy, as a non-medical professional. I am interested not just in the general health delivery mechanisms of conventional medicine; and not just in the knowledge production, products development, methodologies of research, and practices that define what the World Health Organization (WHO) has identified, since the 1970s, as non-conventional medicine (NCM). I am also interested in how these specialized disciplines of health are related to the fields of religious research and practices that speak directly and indirectly to issues of human health, disease, illness, and healthcare. In this sense, healing practices and beliefs about illness are part of a community's wellness system. This system, as Hector Avalos argues, is understood as 'a set of interacting resources, institutions, and strategies that are intended to maintain or restore health in a particular community. Such a system includes, but is not limited to, beliefs about the causes of illness, options available to patients, and the role of governments in healthcare' [33; p 760]. How does this system work? What important religious and social variables and factors contribute to its understanding of, and approach to, disease prevention and treatment, patient–healer relations, patient empowerment and continuing membership in the community? How might information sharing, community mobilizing, support structures, training, attention to belief systems, habits and practices, and environmental factors all contribute to holistic health?

To situate my reflections, I point to the questions of the prophet Jeremiah: 'Is there no balm in Gilead? Is there no healer/physician there? Why then is there no recovery for the daughter of my people?' (Jeremiah 8:22). The issues in Jeremiah's questions are threefold: (1) the basis for understanding and mobilizing the relation between religion and health, both concepts broadly defined; (2) consideration of the active relation between the religious leader and the healer or physician; and (3) the ethical question about the lack of healing for a wounded and hurting community. In other words, I want to use this biblical text to explore the theoretical basis of religion and health, the 'professional' and even institutional partnerships necessary for the implementation of that interdisciplinary work, and the ethical and practical needs and considerations necessary to making healing accessible for those in need. Extrapolating from these musings, I want to pose three framing questions as follows. (a) How are theology, religion, and spirituality historically and/or contemporaneously related to understandings of health, wellness, and healthcare? The fact that some of the most renown medical institutions of research and care are historically tied to religious communities and traditions warrants consideration of intentional (not accidental) kinships between religion and health. (b) What kinds of partnerships and networks could be marshaled and mobilized to address the global disparity in healthcare access and quality treatment? (c) What kinds of ethical and cross-cultural standards and competencies need to be set and implemented to foster creative and productive interdisciplinary approaches to global healthcare, around medicine and religion?

Recognizing the ways in which religion and health may converge and diverge, and conversant of the challenges associated with the very definitions of religion and health [34], I want to examine the above stated questions under two broad frameworks: (1) the theoretical and structural bases for the interdisciplinary work of religion and health; and (2) reflections on the body (physical and communal) as a trope for mobilizing collaborative efforts towards healing. This holistic approach to religion and health assumes a certain anthropological and sociological approach to the human—not as an isolated object of study and scientific or religious observation and theorizing, but as an integrated integer of self and community. One might think here of the complex Bantu-derived notion of Ubuntu as a potent philosophical concept useful not just for communal existence but also for religious and medical healthy existence. To be whole—the biblical analogy here will be the concept of Shalom—requires more than simply a mental or spiritual state of being; it also requires social integration, access to treatment, and sustainable support systems as critically important to the state of healthy being. The contrary is also true: to be sick or ill or unwell is not simply a physical condition but also a psychological and social state of existence. It is in response to these challenges that partnerships in religion and health become potent and enduring.

5.5.2 Religion and health: theoretical and structural underpinning

The constitution of the WHO defines health as 'a state of complete physical, mental and social wellbeing and not merely the absence of disease or infirmity.' Furthermore, the organization sees 'the extension to all peoples of the benefits of medical, psychological and related knowledge' as 'essential to the fullest attainment of health' [35]. This comprehensive vision of health requires a holistic approach to health, one that addresses prevention, diagnosis, and treatment; one that is attentive to conventional medicine as well as NCM. The theoretical underpinning for this approach to health is as follows [36; p 5]:

> The theories and concepts of prevention, diagnosis, improvement and treatment of illness in traditional medicine historically rely on a holistic approach towards the sick individual, and disturbances are treated on the physical, emotional, mental, spiritual and environmental levels simultaneously. As a result, most systems of traditional medicine may use herbal medicines or traditional procedure-based therapies along with certain behavioral rules promoting healthy diets and habits. Holism is a key element of all systems of traditional medicine. Therefore, when reviewing the literature on traditional medicine (both herbal medicines and traditional procedure-based therapies), the theories and concepts of the individual practice of traditional medicine, as well as the cultural background of those involved, must be taken into account.

Arthur Kleinman used a cross-cultural approach to medicine and healing in which 'medicine, like religion', is understood as an 'appropriate subject for linguistic and symbolic analyses' [37; p 30]. Kleinman's argument is also premised on holistic health, attainable through an exploration of healthcare as an integrated system of beliefs, practices, medical professionals, patients, environments, and values. I quote Kleinman at length now [37, p 24] (italics original):

> The single most important concept for the cross-cultural studies of medicine is a radical appreciation that in all societies health care activities are more or less interrelated. Therefore, they need to be studied in a holistic manner as socially organized responses to disease that constitute a special cultural system the *health care system*. In the same way in which we speak of religion or language or kinship as cultural systems, we can view medicine as a cultural system, a system of symbolic meanings anchored in particular arrangements of social institutions and patterns of interpersonal interactions…the health care system, like other cultural systems, integrates the health-related components of society. Patients and healers are basic components of such systems.

The central question then is this: how do religion and faith—as doctrines, beliefs, ritual practices, epistemologies, identity-forming mechanisms, etc—participate in and contribute to this healthcare system? Even with the recognition that the terminology of 'religion' and 'faith' resists easy or singular definition and analyses, the influence of religion and faith on individual and communal approaches to illness and disease, as well as treatment and healing, is undeniable. The persistence of complementary and alternative medicine (CAM) or NCM is indicative of a resurgence, largely since the 1970s, of interest in the age-old question about the correlative and perhaps even a causative relation between religion, ritual, beliefs, and health; and how those relations are conceptualized and methodologies defined for an interdisciplinary approach to health and religion [38].

The *Journal of Religion and Health* emerged from the Academy of Religion and Mental Health. In its first issue (1961) this journal of religion and science included articles by social scientists. In its editorial piece, George Christian Anderson acknowledged the development of specific disciplines of inquiry and research in the Academy, yet also professed the belief that the Academy itself had space for 'a journal attempting to correlate the substance of those disciplines with which the Academy is concerned—namely, medicine, the behavioral sciences, theology, and philosophy—disciplines devoted to healing and the improving of our total health' [38; p 9]. In its multi-disciplinary approach, the journal drew from the fields of anthropology, sociology, psychology, spirituality, and organic medicine to probe and better understand dimensions of health, illness, and wellness, and their relation to organic disturbances and to environmental stress.

The 2010 issue of the *African Health Monitor*, a regional journal of WHO, focused on a decade of work on traditional medicine in Africa. The journal edition examined the theoretical basis of traditional medicine (including its relation to conventional medicine), the methodologies of research and regulation, clinical practices, the use of medicinal plants in the treatment of illnesses (including hypertension), and the need for sustainability through medicinal plant pharmacopeias, policy decisions and implementations, areas of further research and collaboration, etc [40]. In his editorial comments, Luis Gomes Sambo spoke of 'the importance and potential of traditional medicine for the achievement of health for all' [41; p 4]. This potential required the establishment of research programs, the adoption and implementation of public policies that regulate and enhance traditional healthcare, the development of herbal pharmacopoeias, further research on the rich diversity of natural resources, etc. Sambo concluded by urging member nations to 'enhance efforts to train health professionals, health science students and traditional health practitioners in traditional medicine and to foster greater collaboration between the two systems of medicine as a key strategy for institutionalization of traditional medicine into national health systems' [41; p 6].

Similarly, in her introductory essay to a roundtable discussion at Harvard University in 2012 on 'Sacred Healing and Wholeness in Africa and the Americas' Funlayo E Wood wrote [42; p 376]:

> There are, according to a Yoruba tradition, a few major blessings in life—among them, health, wealth, and long life. For many people of African descent —both on the continent and in the diaspora—these three blessings are lacking as African-descended peoples collectively experience worse health outcomes,

more poverty, and shorter active lifespans than their non-African-descended counterparts.

The nature and extent to which health, wealth, and longevity are not only correlative but also causative is an interesting and pertinent subject of inquiry and debate, well beyond the limits of this present essay. But this Yoruba tradition signals that the qualitative indices and mechanisms of life fully lived are best examined and understood as interconnected social mechanisms. Wood posits an 'incontrovertible connection' between these vectors of life-quality, expectancy, and religion among African-descended people and other native peoples (e.g. in the Americas). This connection finds expression or evidence, for example, in the rapidly growing field of CAM that often moves beyond biological paradigms of medicine diagnosis and treatment of the unhealthy body, to include engagement with 'healing techniques' that touch on the religious ('other world') broadly defined. Africana religions thus 'continue to live and thrive by offering their practitioners pathways to wholeness in terms of body, mind, and spirit' [42; pp 377, 378]. Although there are challenges—mechanisms of standardizing, subjectivity of experience, placebo effects, etc—regarding the use of CAMs and NCMs, their popularity and economic power continues in developing and developed countries, and is testament to the need for methodological rigor, regulation, collaborative partnership, and policy building that enhance positive outcomes and curb malpractice or exploitation [43]. Religion and health are, in their most fundamental manifestations and idealistic endeavors, concerned with a common purpose of enhancing human wellbeing in all its dimensions, including sickness prevention, treatment, and palliative care.

5.5.3 Religion, health, and the body

The Hebrew word for 'heart' (*leb*) refers not just to the physical organ of the body but also to the seat of consciousness, deliberation, and moral integrity. In religious (specifically biblical) imagination, the heart attracts special human and divine interest and attention. In the wake of significant political trauma and medical need, Jeremiah's prophetic question about 'healers' in the community (Jeremiah 8:22) eventually construes communal wellness (Shalom) as partly reliant on the function of the heart as an object of divine inscription—that is, as an organ of divine knowledge production and preservation (Jeremiah 31:33). Implementation of the loftiest religious precept (about love for the divine, love for others, and love for oneself) relies on the functioning of the heart: 'You shall love the Lord your God with all your heart...and you shall love your neighbor as yourself.' These understandings of the functioning of the heart are anthropological, religious, and epistemological, not medical. But the texture of meaning associated with the function of the heart in biblical imagination extends into the realm of health and sickness, as we find in the biblical story of Job: unresolved probing of the hidden thoughts and mysteries of the heart is associated with physical bodily sickness and even death (Job 1–2). The link between the physical organ and its symbolic meaning is analogous, yet powerful; it is correlative and even causative. From this analogy between physical and the symbolic health comes such colloquialisms as being 'sick to the stomach' or the sense/feeling that a difficult task gives one 'a headache' or frightened people speaking of almost having a 'heart attack' or upset people described as being 'bent out of shape'. The 'cure' for these unhealthy states of being may be medical or it may be social, cultural, or religious; it certainly may be both [44; p 209].

Research on neuroscience and religion or spirituality is still unfolding and, in some ways, difficult because there is no single standard definition of terms: spirituality and religion have expansive and varied meanings for individuals and for cultures; their effects on the mind and body may range from awe to happiness to hope to mystery; and therefore the subjective experiences associated with religious and spiritual phenomena are difficult to quantify, to verify across time and culture, and therefore to subject to rigorous tests and methodology of repeatability and generalizability. But these difficult methodological and theoretical issues do not warrant retreat from the interdisciplinary work of neuroscience and religion, particularly the physiological aspects of both fields of study. In the fields of psychoneuroendocrinology and psychoneuroimmunology, observations of the autonomic nervous system have shown a number of changes in blood pressure and heart rate resulting from prayer and meditation, as people engage in a *search* for the *sacred* (what an individual perceives 'as divine being, ultimate reality, or ultimate truth') [45; pp 473, 474]. Newberg and Lee explore an intriguing hypothesis: 'If a hypothetical study showed that the practice of meditation results in reductions in cancer rates, it might be valuable to measure the immunological and hormonal status of individuals to determine the physiological basis of the effect' [45; p 474]. It is known that alterations in immune and hormonal functions can affect the brain and vice versa; and so do meditations, as studies in neuroimaging have shown [45; p 477].

From neuroscience to psychoneuroimmunology, the intimate relation between the body and mind is increasingly a topic of rigorous research and theory. Examples include increased endocrine and cardiovascular function in persons who are more socially integrated and benefiting from support groups; the importance of positive and negative beliefs on the functioning of the immune system (e.g. among those suffering from AIDS) and increased chances of survival in metastatic cancer among persons benefiting from strong support systems. All of these lend themselves to the so-called placebo effect: that beliefs (positive or negative) impact how people experience treatment or the effects of medication [44; pp 210, 211].

Studies in clergy health have revealed just how much spiritual leaders suffer from depression, anxiety, and other kinds of non-communicable diseases; but also the critically important role that faith-based organizations (FBOs) play in advancing health education and access in religious institutions [46]. Similarly, Proeschold-Bell *et al* have conducted qualitative research based on a theory of socioecological framework (SEF) that examines five layers of health analyses: intrapersonal that examines an individual's beliefs and characteristics; interpersonal that examines relations between the individual and 'key persons and small social networks' (such as family, friends); community level involving shared identities, experiences, and resources for health; institutional level involving rules, regulations, policies, and ethos that may promote or endanger health; and policy level addressing policies, environments, and structures that impact health. The broadly defined aspects of these layers allow a positing of personal and social relations, as well as exploring the ecologies that connect these layers [47].

There is a rich religious tradition around the question of religion and health from which interpreters embark on a process of 'selective retrieval' [48; p 221] to ground their work, and there is need for deliberate intentionality in framing the question health and wellness and seeking communal partnerships that enhance quality health. A religion that is good only for the health and wellbeing of spirit and the soul, and not for the body is to be pitied (James 2:14–16; Isaiah 58:6–9). As Allen Verhey writes, 'faithful members of religious communities want to live and die and give birth and suffer and care for the suffering with religious integrity, not just with impartial rationality' and this means taking 'theological traditions and religious convictions for medical ethics and religious congregations as communities of moral discourse, character formation, and moral action with respect to questions of medical care' [48; p 222]. The biblical expression 'Balm in Gilead' represents a convergence of religious, political, cultural, and healthcare needs of the community. The expression has been used in African-American scholarship to address the social as well as the psychological effects of racism, particularly depression, among young adults [49]. Also, Lewis V Baldwin used the trope to elucidate the cultural, contextual, communal, and theological threads that defined the life and identity of Martin Luther King Jr, and provide a context for understanding the rugged hope that infused King's work and his repeated reference to the Negro Spiritual, 'There is a Balm in Gilead' [50]. Sara Lawrence Lightfoot's work *Balm in Gilead: Journey of a Healer* is an autobiographical work based on the extraordinary life of her mother—Dr Margaret Lawrence, a medical professional. A sociologist, Lightfoot portrays her mother's struggles to overcome discrimination—around race, gender, class, and geographical region—exploring a life shaped by teaching, preaching, and healing. The title of the book is a reformulation of the biblical prophet and interpreter of society, Jeremiah: 'Is there no balm in Gilead, no healer there?' (Jer. 8:18–22). In an African-American spiritual hymn, this question is answered: 'there is a balm in Gilead, to make the wounded whole' [51].

More than a religious belief, the expression 'Balm in Gilead' is also the name of an international organization whose mission 'is to prevent diseases and to improve the health status of people of the African diaspora by providing support to faith institutions in areas of program design, implementation, and evaluation which strengthens their capacity to deliver programs and services that contribute to the elimination of health disparities' [52]. The professionalization and specialization that define the fields of religious and medical studies afford each individual and community the ability to develop rigorous methodologies of diagnoses and treatment of unhealthy (medical and religious) persons. But professionalization and specialization cannot substitute for, or become alternatives to, the sense of the whole. The challenge is not the distinctiveness of each discipline or its methods, which must continuously be subjected to its standards of rigor, regulation, and ethics; the challenge and the opportunity is the ability to mobilize both fields towards achieving common goals and values, namely, health.

5.5.4 Conclusion

What is the relation between religion and health? How are ritual/religious and medical quarantines similar and/or different? Are medical and religious healing related? To attempt answers to these questions is also to explore the extent to which the disciplines of religion and health (broadly defined) have distinct identities, structured and regulated by specific fields of research, scholarship, practice, regulation, and methodologies of access and service to the larger community. Certainly, both fields generate and deploy significant economic, political, and cultural resources. And both fields have a keen interest in the functioning of the human being (body, mind, spirit), in her/his relation to other humans and to her/his environment (or habitat). But most religions also have a claim about the constitution and the functioning of the human being that is predicated on the reality and active presence of an unquantifiable, mysterious, and yet relatable Being—the divine; that is, not just a generic divine being but a more intimate deity, one that becomes almost kinfolk of the believing individual or community. To inquire of the relation between religion and health, therefore, is to inquire about a relation that is both familiar and unfamiliar. From disease prevention through treatment and palliative care, religion and health are potentially collaborative fields of research. To realize the goal of healing the world, religious and healthcare communities must collaborate to answer some basic but fundamental questions. Put otherwise, to inquire of that relation is to ask mundane and material questions: what does one do with a sick person—body, mind, spirit? What should and does a community do with its sick or unwell members? Why is medical healing so much more than a medical act? And why is religious healing so much more than a religious act? Thus framed, the question of health-related research and practice, very much like that of religion-related research and practice, is not singularly or even primarily an individual endeavor; it is rather a communal one. This understanding of community includes theorizing and relating to the divine as a member of the community; it includes ritualizing and regularizing the experiences and manifestations of that divine presence; and allowing for an element of the unknown that also characterizes the divine, and therefore requires unending striving for fuller and better quality of life for the community.

References

[1] Jha P, Ramasundarahettige C, Landsman V, Rostron B, Thun M, Anderson R N, McAfee T and Peto R 2013 21st-century hazards of smoking and benefits of cessation in the United States *N. Engl. J. Med.* **368** 341–50

[2] Levy D, de Almeida L M and Szklo A 2012 The Brazil SimSmoke policy simulation model: the effect of strong tobacco control policies on smoking prevalence and smoking-attributable deaths in a middle income nation *PLoS Med.* **9** e1001336

[3] Brotherton J M L, Fridman M, May C L, Chappell G, Saville A M and Gertig D M 2011 Early effect of the HPV vaccination programme on cervical abnormalities in Victoria, Australia: an ecological study *Lancet* **377** 2058–92

[4] Torre L A, Siegel R L, Ward E M and Jemal A 2016 Global cancer incidence and mortality rates and trends—an update *Cancer Epidemiol. Biomark. Prevention* **25** doi: 10.1158/1055-9965.EPI-15-0578
[5] Gospodarowicz M 2014 Radiotherapy in global cancer control *Cancer Control* www.cancercontrol.info/cc2014/gospodarowicz/
[6] WHO 2007 Cancer control: knowledge into action *WHO Guide for Effective Programmes* http://apps.who.int/iris/bitstream/10665/43575/1/9241547111_eng.pdf Accessed January 29, 2017
[7] Ullrich A and Miller A 2014 Global response to the burden of cancer: the WHO approach *Am. Soc. Clin. Oncol. Edu.* B **34** e311–5
[8] WHO 2013 *Global Action Plan for the Prevention and Control of Non-Communicable Diseases* 2013–2020 www.who.int/about/licensing/copyright_form/en/index.html Accessed January 29, 2017
[9] Fitzmaurice C, Allen C and Barber R M *et al* 2016 Global, regional, and national cancer incidence, mortality, years of life lost, years lived with disability, and disability-adjusted life-years for 32 cancer groups, 1990 to 2015 *JAMA Oncol.* **388** 1459–544
[10] International Agency for Research on Cancer (GLOBOCAN) 2012 *Estimated Cancer Incidence, Mortality, and Prevalence Worldwide in 2012* http://globocan.iarc.fr/Pages/fact_sheets_population.aspx Accessed January 15, 2017
[11] Thun M J, DeLancey J O, Center M M, Jemal A and Ward E M 2010 The global burden of cancer: priorities for prevention *Carcinogenesis* **31** 100–10
[12] Colditz G, Dejong W, Hunter D, Trichopoulos D and Willett W 1996 Harvard Report on Cancer Prevention. Volume 1: Causes of human cancer *Cancer Causes Control* 7 Suppl. 1 S3-59
[13] Harvard Men's Health Watch 2009 The 10 commandments of cancer prevention *Harvard Health Publications* April www.health.harvard.edu/newsletter_article/The-10-commandments-of-cancer-prevention Accessed January 31, 2017
[14] Sloan F A and Gelband H 2007 Cancer causes and risk factors and the elements of cancer control *Cancer Control Opportunities in Low- and Middle-Income Countries* ed F A Sloan and H Gelband (Washington, DC: National Academies Press) chapter 2
[15] WHO 2013 *WHO Report on the Global Tobacco Epidemic* http://apps.who.int/iris/bitstream/10665/85380/1/9789241505871_eng.pdf Accessed January 31, 2017
[16] WHO 2016 *Prevalence of Tobacco Smoking*
[17] Sreeramareddy C T, Pradhan P M and Sin S 2012 Prevalence, distribution, and social determinants of tobacco use in 30 sub-Saharan African countries *BMC Med.* **380** 2224–60
[18] De Pergola G, Silvestris F 2013 Obesity as a major risk factor for cancer *J. Obesity* **2013** 291546
[19] Bagnardi Vincenzo, Blangiardo Marta, Vecchia Carlo La and Corrao Giovanni 2017 *Alcohol Consumption and the Risk of Cancer* https://pubs.niaaa.nih.gov/publications/arh25-4/263-270.htm Accessed January 31, 2017
[20] Plummer M, de Martel C, Vignat J, Ferlay J, Bray F and Franceschi S 2016 Global burden of cancers attributable to infections in 2012: a synthetic analysis *Lancet Global Health* **4** e609–16
[21] Sloan F and Gelband H (ed) 2007 *Cancer Control Opportunities in Low- and Middle-Income* (Washington, DC: National Academies Press)
[22] V Foundation 2017 *Remembering Jim* www.jimmyv.org/about/remembering-jim/
[23] BrainyQuote www.brainyquote.com/quotes/quotes/j/jimvalvano358457.html Accessed June 23, 2017
[24] Associated Press 2006 Mutombo gives $15 million for hospital in Congo *ESPN* 14 August www.espn.co.uk/nba/news/story?id=2549321

[25] OECD *Harnessing the Skills of Migrants and Diaspora to Foster Development: Policy Options*
Bradatan, Popan and Melton *Transnationality as a Fluid Social Identity*
Faist *Towards Transnational Studies: World Theories, Transnationalisation and Changing Institutions*
[26] World Bank *African Diaspora Key to the Continents Development*
World Bank *Diaspora Remittances Must Open the Door to Financial Inclusion*
Bodomo *African Diaspora Remittances Are Better than Foreign Aid Funds*
Kemegue, Owusu-Sekyere and van Eyden *Harnessing Remittances through Formal Channels for Development in Sub-Saharan Africa*
[27] Clemens, Özden and Rapoport *Migration and Development Research Is Moving Far Beyond Remittances*
OECD *Harnessing the Skills of Migrants and Diaspora to Foster Development: Policy Options*
Brinkerhoff *Creating an Enabling Environment for Diasporas' Participation in Homeland Development*
[28] Kshetri *The Diaspora as a Change Agent on Entrepreneurship-Related Institutions in Sub-Saharan Africa*
Alex-Assensoh *African Americans, African Immigrants and Homeland-Diaspora Development in Africa*
Davies *African Diasporas, Development and the Politics of Context*
[29] Norman C 1981 *The God That Limps: Science and Technology in the Eighties* (New York: W. W. Norton)
[30] Dolmage J 2006 'Breath upon us an even flame': Hephaestus, history and the body of rhetoric *Rhetoric Rev.* **25** 119-40
[31] Djibril Tamsir Niane 1994 *Sundiata: An Epic of Old Mali. transl.* ed G D Pickett (Harlow: Longman)
[32] Mary Douglas 1966 *Purity and Danger: An Analysis of the Concepts of Pollution and Taboo* (New York: Praeger)
[33] Avalos H 2007 Health care *The New Interpreter's Dictionary of the Bible*vol 2 ed K D Sakenfeld *et al* (Nashville, TN: Abingdon)
Avalos H 1999 *Health Care and the Rise of Christianity* (Peabody MA: Hendrickson)
[34] Matthew T Bergsagel-Braley 2014 Global health after Pentecost: toward theological reflection as a religious health asset *Christian J. Global Health* **1** 48-62
Jeff Levin 2009 'And let us make us a name': reflections on the future of the religion and health field *J. Religion Health* **48** 125-45
[35] WHO www.who.int/about/mission/en/
[36] WHO 2000 *General Guidelines for Methodologies on Research and Evaluation of Traditional Medicine* (Geneva: WHO)
[37] Arthur Kleinman 1980 *Patients and Healers in the Context of Culture: An Exploration of the Borderland between Anthropology, Medicine, and Psychiatry* (Berkeley, CA: University of California Press)
[38] For more see; Kottow Michael H 1992 Classical medicine v alternative medical practices *J. Med. Ethics* **18** 18-22
Franck Linda, Chantler Cyril, Dixon Michael and Colquhoun David 2007 Should NICE evaluate alternative and comparative medicine? *Br. Med.* J **334** 506-7
[39] George Christian Anderson 1961 Editorial *J. Religion Health* **1** 9–11

[40] WHO 2010 Decade of African traditional medicine (2000–2010) *African Health Monitor Special Edition* #13, August

[41] Luis Gomes Sambo 2010 The decade of African traditional medicine: progress so far *African Health Monitor* #13, August, 4–6

[42] Funlayo E Wood 2013 Sacred healing and wholeness in Africa and the Americas *J. Africana Religions* **1**

[43] Emmanuel Kabengele Mpinga *et al* 2013 Traditional/alternative medicines and the right to health: key elements for a convention on global health *Health Human Rights* **15** 46–54

[44] Patricia Forsarelli 2002 Fearfully wonderfully made: the interconnectedness of body–mind–spirit *J. Religion Health* **41**

[45] Newberg Andrew B and Lee Bruce Y 2005 The neuroscientific study of religious and spiritual phenomena: or why god doesn't use biostatistics *Zygon* **40**

[46] Webb Benjamin, Bopp Melissa and Fallon Elizabeth A 2013 A qualitative study of faith leaders' perceptions of health and wellness *J. Religion Health* **52** 235–46

[47] Proeschold-Bell Rae Jean, LeGrand Sara, James John, Wallace Amanda, Adams Christopher and Toole David 2011 A theoretical model of the holistic health of United Methodist clergy *J. Religion Health* **50** 703

[48] Allen D Verhey 1990 Talking of God: but with whom? *Hastings Center Rep.* **20** 221

[49] Ellison Christopher G, Musick Marc A and Henderson Andrea K 2008 Balm in Gilead: racism, religious involvement, and psychological distress among African-American young adults *J. Sci. Study Religion* **47** 291–301

[50] Lewis V Baldwin 1991 *There is a Balm in Gilead: The Cultural Roots of Martin Luther King Jr* (Minneapolis, MN: Fortress) p 5

[51] Sara Lawrence Lightfoot 1988 *Balm in Gilead: Journey of a Healer* (Reading, MA: Addison-Wesley)

[52] Balm in Gilead http://www.balmingilead.org/mission Accessed January 14, 2017

Chapter 6

Frequently asked questions in global oncology

Omoruyi Credit Irabor, Paul L Nguyen and Wilfred Ngwa

6.1 FAQs on global oncology care

6.1.1 Cobalt machines versus linear accelerators: which one is better in global oncology?

Editor's notes:

Over 50% of cancer patients need radiation therapy [1]. In the Lancet Oncology Commission report on expanding global access to radiotherapy, Atun *et al* provide compelling evidence that investment in radiotherapy not only enables treatment of large numbers of cancer cases to save lives, but also brings positive economic benefits. The Lancet Oncology Commission report [1] calls for expansion of access to radiotherapy, targeting at least one cancer center in each low and middle income country (LMIC) to have radiotherapy services by 2020, and a 25% increase in radiotherapy treatment capacity by 2025. A big first question these days to consider when procuring a radiotherapy machine for an LMIC is whether to buy a cobalt machine or a linear accelerator (LINAC).

LINACs use high frequency electromagnetic waves to accelerate charged particles such as electrons to high energies for use during radiotherapy. The high-energy electron itself can be used for treating superficial tumors or it can be made to strike a tungsten target to produce x-rays for treating deep-seated tumors. Meanwhile typical Cobalt machines use a Cobalt-60 gamma ray as the source of radiation. The decision whether to purchase a Cobalt machine versus a LINAC has been a major cause for intellectual debate within the radiation oncology community. It is one of the most frequently asked questions for LMIC looking to include radiotherapy in their cancer control plans. The following sections answer this question from different perspectives.

doi:10.1088/978-0-7503-1359-9ch6

Perspective of Professor Twalib Ngoma (Former Director of the Ocean Road Cancer Institute and leading African clinical oncologist (medical oncology and radiation oncology))

When I was setting up radiotherapy services in Tanzania in the 1980s I choose a cobalt-60 machine, in spite of the fact that I knew that LINACs have several advantages over cobalt-60 machines, such as the ability to create very high energy beams, with the edges of the beams much more sharply defined than those of a cobalt machine. LINACs allow additional precision in dose delivery, the capability to produce electron beams that are of particular value in treating superficial lesions, and a dose rate that can be regulated as opposed to that of cobalt, which is determined by the amount of cobalt source in the machine and cannot be regulated. The factors which influenced my decision to choose cobalt as opposed to LINAC are: they are not as robust as cobalt machines in our environment; they require technical maintenance support not available in Tanzania; they require a stable electricity power supply, which is a rare commodity in Tanzania; and LINACs also require trained physicists/technicians to operate them. At that time Tanzania had no physicists. Another consideration was upfront cost, although over a period of ten years taking source replacement into account the cost of a 6 MV LINAC and that of a cobalt machine are not significantly different. If you ask me the major factor for choosing a cobalt machine instead of a LINAC at that time, the answer is *lack of physicists*.

Perspective from India, by Sridhar P Susheela and Swaroop Revannasiddaiah. Reproduced from 'Rekindling the immortal debate—telecobalt versus linear accelerator' (2015 *Cancer Control* **11** 243–244)

> The telecobalt versus linear-accelerator debate often drags into a 'which is superior–which is inferior' argument, and that leads to an undue focusing upon the shortcomings of technology. This in turn takes the impetus away from the ponderings over 'potential and possibilities'. But in the broad perspective, there should be no existential threat to either the telecobalt or the linear accelerator, because of the other—there is room for both to co-exist!...the linear accelerator, being endowned with better beam characteristics can do a lot more things which cannot be done with a telecobalt...However, speaking from the perspective of the average Indian radiotherapy facility, the requirements are different and rather dire. The ability to cater to a very large number of patients is one thing a linear accelerator cannot be expected to reliably satisfy all year round. Then, given the beaurocratic hurdles that government treatment facilities often face, it can be said that meeting the financial costs involved in the maintenance and running of a linear accelerator cannot always be ensured, and this too can contribute to down-time. There have been many instances wherein linear accelerators remain unused for months—and at times years—for expensive reasons such as klystron failure, waveguide damage, and the such. Without a doubt, linear accelerator is technically more advanced, and more versatile with regards to the add-on capabilities. But there are a few practical

advantages with the tele-cobalt which cannot be provided by the linear accelerator. These advantages of the telecobalt are very much of relevance in the Indian scenario, with special reference to the financially challenged government institutions…In conclusion, instead of thinking about getting rid of the telecobalt, it would be very pragmatic to retain the old trusted warhorse of the Indian radiotherapy scenario, and the addition of the multi-leaf collimator would enable wonderful possibilities. The addition of the MLC would in no way make the telecobalt equivalent to a linear accelerator, but after all, who is doing a comparison here? A telecobalt machine with an in-built ability to provide shaped-field radiotherapy would be good for the sea of cancer patients in India. That is all that matters.

Perspective of Massoud Samiei (Independent international expert collaborating with the IAEA, WHO, IARC, UICC, Oxford University, and INCTR). Reproduced from 'Challenges of making radiotherapy accessible in developing countries' (2013 *Cancer Control* **8** 85–96)

Cobalt-60 units have traditionally been considered the more robust workhorses to place in new cancer clinics in developing countries. Their cost is lower, and they are easier to operate for treatment delivery, planning, and maintenance. However, cobalt machines have become much more sophisticated and their prices have increased. Also the cost of cobalt-60 sources is much higher and there are heightened security concerns after the 9/11 incident making the transport and return of spent sources more complicated. Some LINAC manufacturers have also provided incentives like participating in the investment at country level through joint ventures (some good examples are in Peru, Turkey and Vietnam). As a result, there are already many developing countries in Asia and Latin America (and a few in Africa) who are operating LINACs, though with some maintenance issues. On the other hand, a few manufacturers have recently placed on the market small, single-energy LINACs (4–6 MeV) at lower overall costs. Others are following suit. Thus, for the LMIC governments or investors, the choices could be soon roughly comparable when combining initial capital and future recurring costs between cobalt and LINACs. It is clear that the current and emerging need for teletherapy units in developing countries cannot be met by cobalt machines alone. The selection of equipment will depend on the country's radiotherapy experience and its financial and technical capacity and the available workforce. For cobalt machines, which have a useful life of 20 years, in addition to their increased initial cost, the main issue today is the need to replace the cobalt-60 source every 5–6 years (about US$150 000), requiring often disposal of the old sources at very high costs (US$250 000 to US$350 000, save prior arrangements during procurement). For the cobalt-60 source, special authorization and licensing is required from other countries in transit, unless the supplier is able to use international routes and direct transport means. For LINACs, which can be operated for 10–12 years before replacement, the capital cost is still high and their commissioning, operation, training, QA programs and maintenance requirements are more complex and costly. For most LMICs, having operated and used cobalts for a number of years, a mix-choice is probably the right approach when resources are available.

Perspective of the International Atomic Energy Agency (IAEA)

According to an article in 2016 titled 'A balanced approach to radiotherapy: integrating cobalt-60 machines and linear accelerators treatment' [1] the IAEA also has provided perspective in answering the question of cobalt-60 versus LINACs.

The guidance or perspective provided by the IAEA highlights the most important factors to be considered when deciding on the type of radiotherapy equipment to invest in for cancer treatment [1]:

> 'It is important to evaluate each aspect of the equipment choice, first of all the anticipated clinical benefits to patients but also the management of the technology over time to ensure that it will deliver consistently safe and effective treatment,' said Ahmed Meghzifene, Head of the Dosimetry and Medical Radiation Physics section at the IAEA. 'If not correctly handled and maintained, radiotherapy equipment may deliver non-optimal treatments to patients and in extreme situations may cause harm.'

Factors highlighted include:

1. *Extra costs.* Experts indicate that the cost of operating teletherapy machines goes beyond the purchase costs. There is need for treatment planning which requires diagnostic equipment such as computed tomography scanners, patient set-up devices and so forth. These extra costs need to be carefully considered.
2. *Personnel requirements.* Because of the higher level of sophistication of radiotherapy machines Medical Physicists, engineers, and other operating personnel must be properly trained. These personnel requirements need to be taken into account. Stakeholders have to consider whether to set up local training programs or send them abroad.

According to May Abdel-Wahab, the Director for the Division of Human Health at IAEA, there is no standard answer to the choice of radiotherapy equipment. Such a choice should be made after careful analysis that takes into account both the technological characteristics of the machines but also the local infrastructure, the evaluation of maintenance requirements, affordability, and the available trained personnel.

Perspective from the Editors

According to global health experts such as Jacob Van Dyk, there are a number of criteria to take into account when making a decision comparing radiation therapy machines. These include the radiation beam characteristics, such as beam edge sharpness, energy, scatter conditions or dose uniformity, contour or inhomogeneity corrections, dose to bone, machine characteristics (e.g. source to surface distance, dose rate, radioactive source versus x-rays), service or maintenance issues, safety considerations (e.g. radiation protection, pacemaker concerns), and cost considerations. From our perspective based on interactions with many stakeholders, we have adopted a neutral position and see the Global Health Catalyst (GHC) as a platform for facilitating meetings between LMIC stakeholders and the different industry actors to allow them develop an optimal solution for each individual case.

6.1.2 What manufacturer or pharmaceutical company should I choose?

Another FAQ is the choice of industry stakeholder. For most LMICs, industry stakeholders such as radiotherapy manufacturers are often located far from the purchasing country, most commonly in Europe or North America. Factors to be considered include transportation costs and maintenance issues, e.g. warranty. The choice of industry stakeholder should consider warranty and maintenance contracts. Once the warranty expires, or if it does not adequately cover the costs, cancer centers are forced to leave a machine non-operational, due to insufficient funds to support maintenance and upkeep or source replacement. It is therefore crucial that a maintenance contract be a factor in the choice of industry stakeholder and whether the supplier has established service centers close to the LMIC center. If not, adequate local maintenance staff trained by the supplier could help to reduce costs associated with long-distance travel between supplier and the LMIC center.

6.1.3 Once you have decided on a LINAC or cobalt machine, what do you have to do before the machine is installed and ready to use in treatment?

Answer with Perspective from Tanzania by Professor Twalib Ngoma (Former Director of Ocean Road Cancer Institute and Chair of Department of Clinical Oncology, Muhimbili University of Health and Allied Sciences, Tanzania)

After the decision to buy a machine was made and we had the money to buy the machine, I did the following:

1. Hired architects to prepare drawings for the bunker and bidding documents for contractors who will build the bunker.
2. Requested for approval of the drawings from the Tanzania Atomic Energy Commission (TAEC) and International Atomic Energy Agency (IAEA).
3. Advertised a tender for competitive bidding for the building of bunker project.
4. Involved TAEC and IAEA from the beginning to the end of the building project.
5. Sent an official request to the IAEA in Vienna through the TAEC to give us technical support in the procurement, transportation, installation, and commissioning of the cobalt machine.
6. Requested for IAEA fellowships to train personnel such as physicists and radiotherapy technologists

6.1.4 How do radiotherapy incorporation and the supply process work in LMICs?

The procurement process is a vital element of equitable radiotherapy accessibility. The WHO defines this process as 'the acquisition of property, plant, equipment, goods, works or services through purchase, hire, lease, rental or exchange', which includes 'all actions from planning and forecasting, identification of needs, sourcing, and solicitation of offers, evaluation of proposals, review, and award of contracts, contracting and all phases of contract administration until delivery of the goods, the end of a contract, or the useful life of an asset.' In specialties like radiation oncology, where procurement includes installation and commissioning, the process is better termed as 'technology incorporation' [2]. Using the workflow detailed in a WHO technical manual on technology incorporation as prototype, the flowchart for a standard radiotherapy incorporation and management procedure spans through a planning phase, acquisition phase, utilization phase, and disposal (see figure 6.1).

In figure 6.1, divisions I, II, and III, mark the 'radiotherapy planning stage'. Divisions IV and V are the 'radiotherapy acquisition phase', while divisions VI, VII, and VIII mark the 'radiotherapy utilization phase' of the radiotherapy management cycle, which is just prior to decommissioning, then disposal (IX) and replacement. The supply side involves the conception and delivery of radiotherapy technology and innovation to the hands of end-users in a supply chain model. Radiotherapy equipment supplies in LMICs are usually by direct procurement, donation, or lease. Due to the complexity and safety requirement of radiotherapy and nuclear isotopes, the role of radiotherapy suppliers also cuts through various phases of the radiotherapy management cycle, including planning of service deliveries, business negotiations with purchasers, workforce development, installations, maintenance,

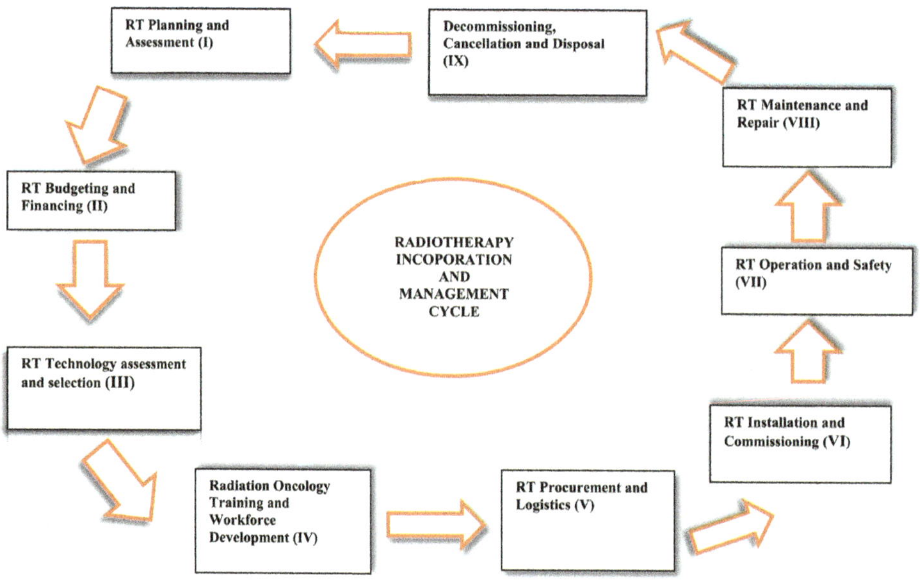

Figure 6.1. Radiotherapy incorporation and management cycle.

and disposal of isotope sources. Thus, radiotherapy suppliers stand out as stakeholders whose inputs, market access, technical expertise, and global health inclinations immensely influence the success and limitations of global radiation oncology.

Indeed, poor practices in radiotherapy acquisition, such as equipment supply with no quality assurance manual or replacement plan, have been known to impede progress in global cancer care and have resulted in the unnecessary waste of already limited financial resource in some LMICs. The goal and criteria for measuring supply chain performance are yet unspecified for global radiation oncology. However, based on standards of practice for healthcare supplies, a strong radiotherapy supply chain is expected to satisfy the following: cost-effectiveness, appropriate quality and technology adoption, on-time delivery of equipment and isotope sources and repair services, expected quantity, satisfactory installations and training, active warranty for every radiotherapy procurement, adequate maintenance and replacement plan of radiotherapy source and equipment, and a transparent and trustworthy service. To achieve this goal and for transparency purposes, public procurement of radiotherapy equipment is supposed to be carried out according to the principles of International Competitive Bidding (ICB). The ICB is a bidding process that involves eight major steps, from the choice of what equipment or structure is required, up to the evaluation and quality assurance process (figure 6.2).

6.1.5 What are your current challenges in designing equipment packages that are affordable and suitable for LMICs?

One market shaping approach to finding a lasting solution to the gross equipment shortage, first initiated by the IAEA in 2010, was the bid on manufacturers of radiotherapy devices to design equipment packages that are more affordable and suitable for developing countries. Major radiotherapy design innovation has been made in recent years, aimed at treating a larger number of patients more quickly with better clinical outcomes, accompanied by higher reliability and 'uptime'. This innovation is not limited to the developing world but relevant to it, as radiotherapy centers in LMICs can (in principle) operate their machines 2–3 shifts per day, treating up to 60–70 patients per day, and up to 6000 patients per year. Accompanying planning software establishes baseline quality and reduces the risk of error, and shortens planning and treatment times further. However, it is hard to tell if LMICs are willing to accept these innovations.

According to one leading manufacturer, Dow Wilson (President and CEO Varian Medical Systems; see section 4.1 for full interview): 'Ministers and public health decision-makers in LMICs indicate their preference for a range of radiotherapy machines, linked often to a 'hub and spoke' cancer network with higher-end machines clustered in 'hub' academic teaching hospitals. Often they do not want even low energy LINACs, despite the apparent better 'fit' with their environments. As compared to diagnostics—where the benefits of small, mobile diagnostics are clear—it is not certain that LMIC decision-makers favor such development directions.' Clearly, one challenge to such an innovation is acceptance.

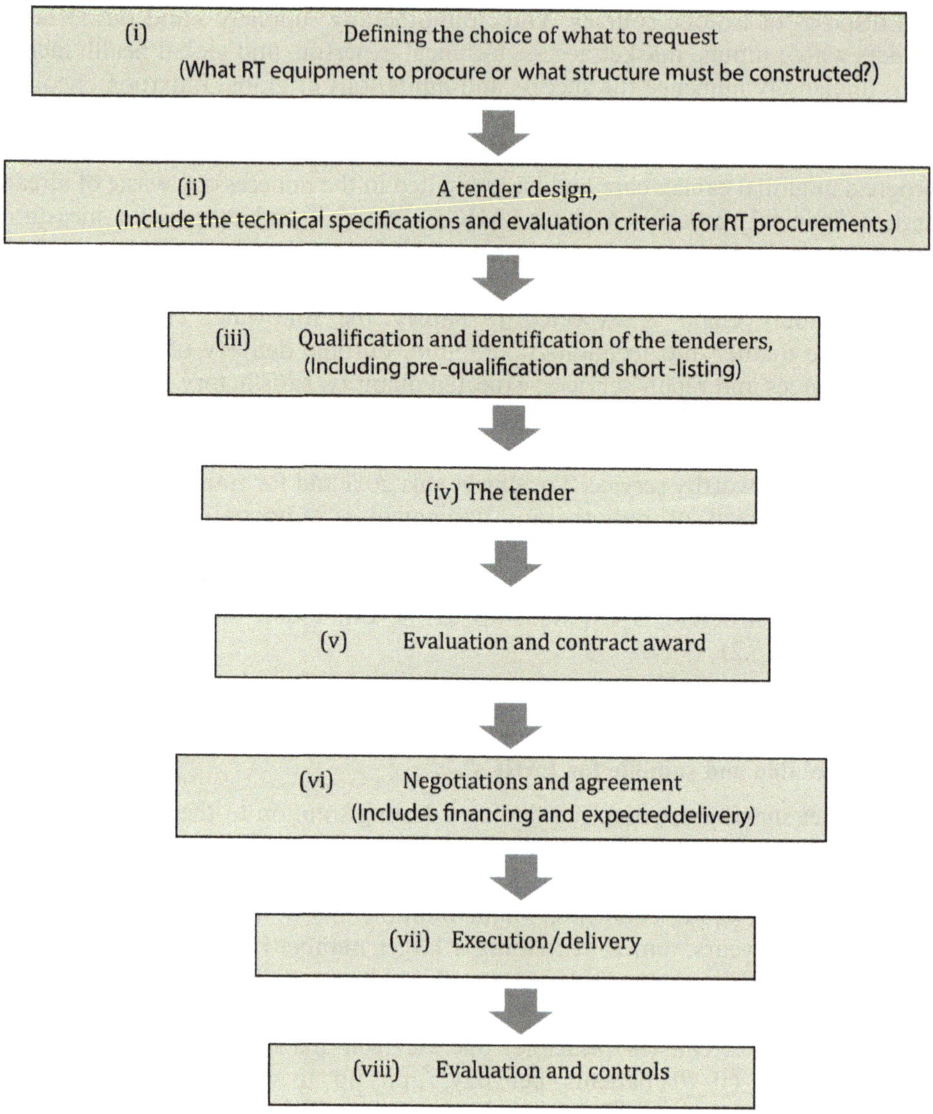

Figure 6.2. International competitive bidding framework for radiotherapy procurement.

6.1.6 What are some low-cost radiotherapy innovations for low resource countries?

While acceptance remains an issue, specific low-cost innovations are worth mentioning. The UNIQUE™, designed by Varian Medical Systems, is a comprehensive and cost-effective low-energy radiotherapy system with image-guidance and RapidArc treatment capabilities. Varian now offers a version of this solution without the RapidArc technology or image-guidance software with a more basic yet upgradeable platform, affordable for cancer centers in low resource settings. The Elekta

Compact™ is a cost-effective solution which constitutes a flexible yet affordable compact LINAC, with a small footprint and a cost-effective design. The operation of this system is relatively simple and it is reliable, allowing more patients to be treated quickly and effectively. With its modular design, upgrades and new functions and features can be added easily, making it a robust stand-alone solution for radiation therapy. TeamBest designed the Therathron, a cobalt-60 based EBRT, known for its significantly low initial investment, simplicity, and reduced downtime. In addition, the Theratron® Equinox™ operates with standard electrical power and does not need a special cooling system, thereby reducing the operational cost of the unit. Theratrons have been upgraded with the latest intensity modulated radiotherapy (IMRT), image-guided radiotherapy (IGRT), and stereotactic radiosurgery (SRS) technologies.

A useful reference is Atun R *et al* 2015 Expanding global access to radiotherapy *Lancet Oncol.* **16** 1153–86.

6.2 FAQ on global oncology research

6.2.1 How do I get funding for research in global oncology?

Chapter 2 includes a lecture by the National Cancer Institute on opportunities for funding. In general the National Cancer Institute for Global Health has a listing of funding opportunities as does Fogarty International in the USA. Fogarty International also has a listing of funding opportunities by other funding agencies. Outside the USA, most developed countries, such as Canada, Germany, UK, France, Japan, Italy, Netherlands, and so forth, have national funding agencies that support cancer research. A directory of national and international cancer institutes, centers and organizations can be found on the website www.cancerindex.org/clinks7.htm. International directories of foundations can be found on the website http://grantspace.org/tools/knowledge-base. The Grantsmanship center also provides a list of international funding sources: www.tgci.com/international-funding-sources. Some examples of global oncology funders are listed in table 6.1.

6.2.2 Who is doing what in global oncology research?

The global cancer project map is useful resource to answer this question: http://globalonc.org/Projects/global-cancer-project-map/.

6.2.3 How do I participate in clinical trials?

The National Cancer Institute provides a platform for finding clinical trials: www.cancer.gov/about-cancer/treatment/clinical-trials/search. The Radiation Therapy Oncology Group (RTOG) also has a listing of clinical trials. The RTOG is a national clinical cooperative group for the purpose of conducting radiation therapy research and cooperative clinical investigations www.rtog.org/ClinicalTrials/ProtocolTable.aspx.

Table 6.1. Some examples of global oncology funders.

Funding agency	Website and comments
Abbott Fund	http://abbottfund.org Supports non-communicable diseases and HIV/AIDS in underserved regions of the world.
Abbvie Foundation	www.bms.com/foundation/ Funds cancer relief in Central and Eastern Europe and provides grants for HIV/AIDS treatment and prevention in sub-Saharan Africa.
Boren Awards	www.borenawards.org/ Supports USA students to study or have international experience abroad.
Doris Duke Charitable Foundation	www.ddcf.org/ Provides funding for medical research and strengthening health systems.
European Commission	https://ec.europa.eu/research/health/ Funds international collaborations in cancer research.
Izumi Foundation	http://izumi.org/ Funds programs that improve health in developing countries.
European Association for Cancer Research	www.eacr.org/travel-fellowships Provides opportunities for early-career scientists to advance their research including travel fellowships.
Izumi Foundation	http://izumi.org/ Funds programs that improve health in developing countries.
Merck Company Foundation	www.msdresponsibility.com/our-giving/ The charitable arm of the pharmaceutical company focuses its grantmaking on building healthcare worker capacity in developing countries.
Seed Global Health	http://seedglobalhealth.org/ Supports new generations of US health professionals to serve as global health educators and work within countries facing critical human healthcare resource shortages.
Welcome Trust (UK)	https://wellcome.ac.uk/ Provides funding for biomedical science, population health, product development, and applied research.
World Cancer Research Fund International	www.wcrf.org/int/research-we-fund Funds research on the effects of diet, nutrition, body composition, and physical activity on cancer prevention and survival.

6.3 FAQ on global oncology education

6.3.1 Where can I get training?

Many of the leading cancer organizations in the world provide training opportunities, e.g. African Organization for Research and Training in Cancer, American Society for Clinical Oncology, European Society for Clinical Oncology, the World Health

Organization, and other societies highlighted in chapter 1. Most global health departments or institutions in the USA and Europe also provide training opportunities

6.3.2 Where can I get scholarships?

Many of the organizations that provide training also offer scholarships. Developed countries also have programs that provide international scholarships, e.g. the Fulbright Scholarships, DAAD Scholarships, and Humboldt Foundation Fellowships. Fogarty International also has a good list of opportunities.

6.4 Other frequently asked questions

6.4.1 What are the ways to prevent cancer?

The Dana Farber Cancer Institute recently published '10 Evidence-Based Cancer Prevention Tips', shown in figure 6.3. Some 'best buys' in cancer prevention were also discussed in the lecture from the American Cancer Society in chapter 5.

6.4.2 How can the diaspora participate in global oncology?

Chapter 5 discusses some ways for the diaspora to participate that were identified during the 2016 Harvard Global Health Catalyst (GHC) summit. Some of these ways include advocacy, cancer education and awareness, cancer prevention, crowdfunding research, online education, and telemedicine.

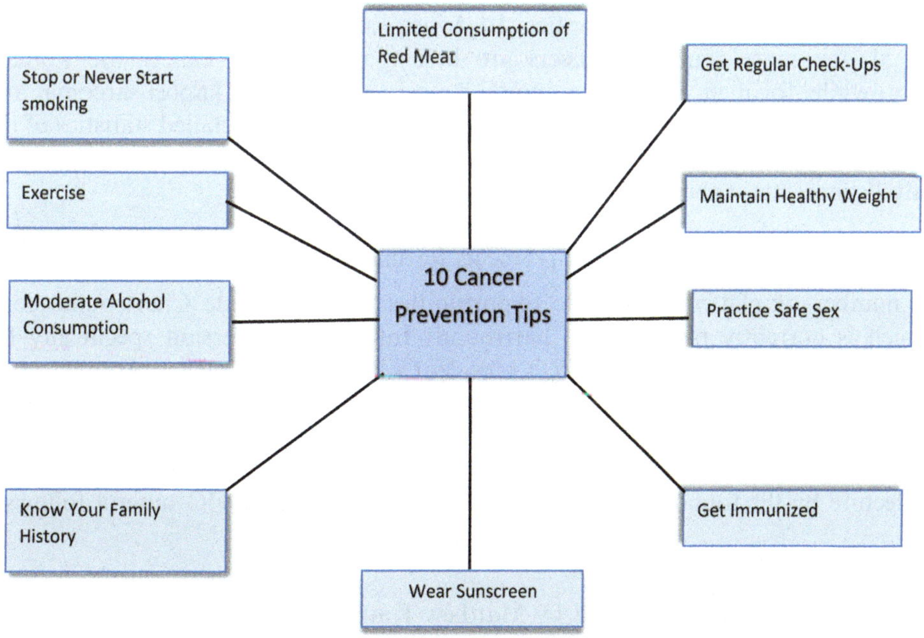

Figure 6.3. 10 evidence-based cancer prevention tips. Reproduced with permission from [3].

6.4.3 How can I participate in global oncology?

The GHC summit is a great opportunity to connect and plug-in to opportunities for global oncology. A number of recent publications coming out of the GHC summit at Harvard address this question comprehensively, including for people who want to participate in global health but have little time or do not want to travel. Below are some publications in this light:

- Ngwa W *et al* 2015 The potential for information and communication technologies to catalyze global collaborations in radiation oncology *Int. J. Radiat. Oncol. Biol. Phys.* **91** 444–7
- Ngwa W and Ngoma T 2016 *Emerging Models for Global Health in Radiation Oncology* (Bristol: IOP Publishing)
- Ngwa W *et al* 2016 Closing the cancer divide through Ubuntu: information and communication technology-powered models for global radiation oncology *Int. J. Radiat. Oncol. Biol. Phys.* **94** 440–9

6.4.4 What are the greatest challenges to global health?

Key challenges identified are poor healthcare systems: lack of infrastructure, e.g. radiotherapy treatment facilities; affordability; little research or research funding; the dearth in human capacity to address the growing cancer burden; and a lack of country cancer control plans. The book *Closing the Cancer Divide* (2012; Cambridge, MA: Harvard University Press), edited by Felicia Knaul *et al*, is a good resource.

6.4.5 What are the priority cancers to address in global oncology?

Each region has different priorities. In Africa, according to different publictions [4, 5], the most common cancers are breast and cervical cancer for women. Meanwhile, for men, the most common cancers are prostate, kaposi sarcoma, and liver cancers. The American Cancer Society cancer atlas has detailed statistics of the priority or most common cancers in different regions. The map can be accessed here: http://canceratlas.cancer.org/the-burden/.

6.4.6 How can I get help or find protocols for management of individual cancers?

A number of platforms provide opportunities. These include Chartrounds.com, which is currently planning a Chartrounds International version specifically for LMICs, highlighted in the ASTRO president's lecture in chapter 3. Another good platform for getting help in general is the Global Health Delivery Project at Harvard (www.globalhealthdelivery.org/). For global radiation oncology a good platform is Radiation Nation, a platform for collaborative conversations in radiation oncology. A lecture by the founder of Radiation Nation given at the GHC summit follows.

6.4.7 What is Radiation Nation?

Radiation Nation was founded by Matthew Katz in the early 2000s as a collaborative community for sharing knowledge in radiation medicine. Its goal is to improve cancer care through discussion of clinically relevant aspects in radiation oncology.

Specific areas of interest include patient education, collaborative medical practice, and improving quality and safety. The initiative ensures a collaborative approach to sharing for all involved in the use of radiation medicine: patients, caregivers, and medical professionals. Although radiation oncology is very technology-driven, the purpose of those technologies remains healing and caring. Its fundamental guiding principles remain the same as medicine in general. The Radiation Nation website aims to be a resource to lessen suffering and enhance health. In defining the philosophy behind the initiative, Mathew Katz states:

> Expertise is essential but never perfect. We value the contributions of academic and community healthcare professionals, patients, caregivers, and anyone else interested enough to share. All opinions, whether you're an expert or know little, are respected and valuable when the goal is to improve care.

Community guidelines include: (i) respect, both in clinical practice and online conversation; (ii) transparency; (iii) patient privacy, Radiation Nation is HIPPA

Table 6.2. Radiation Nation resources.

Clinical trials	The Radiation Nation web-page provides links to all clinical trials in oncology going on worldwide, which help scholars keep abreast with ongoing research in their field.
Decision aids	Decision aids provided include the breast cancer decision aid, lung cancer decision aid, and prostate cancer decision aid.
Directories	(Currently being developed)
Radiation resources	Resources include: • Clinical practice guidelines • Safety, quality improvement, and research • Advocacy and patient education • Health communications (blogs) • Radiation communities • Organizations: Cancer care • Organizations: Radiation oncology • Organizations: Radiation therapy/radiography • Organizations: Dosimetry and medical physics • Organizations: Nursing
Patient education resources	Each participant can learn differently based upon language, literacy, and cognitive style. Radiation Nation provides links and resources to help individualize patient education. Thus, clinicians can review these before recommending them to patients, because there are likely to be differences to their usual practice of explaining to patients.
Radiation safety resources	Radiation Nation aid with links to radiation safety resources in: • Diagnostic imaging • Environmental exposure • Radioisotopes and radiation measurement • International Atomic Energy Agency (IAEA) • Communicating risk

compliant in its terms of use; and (iv) collaborative. Currently, Radiation Nation is designed to allow multiple authors to post articles under a variety of topics. On any given piece, community members can share their experience, knowledge, and questions by commenting. Participants can also share on Facebook, Twitter, and other social media platforms. Radiation Nation resources include clinical trials, decision aids, directories, radiation resources, patient education resources, and radiation safety resources, as shown in table 6.2.

Current challenges of Radiation Nation are in access and a lack of awareness, which has resulted in limited collaboration or contributions from some regions of the world. Limitations in access have to do with connectivity issues, which range from low bandwidth, slow internet connections, and high internet service charges in LMICs. Due to a lack of awareness, web traffic is relatively small, even from countries such as Nigeria or South Africa where daily internet usage hovers around 67% and 57%, respectively. Radiation Nation is currently partnering with the GHC at Harvard Medical School and the African Organization for Research and Training in Cancer (AORTIC) to implement a formal e-learning platform that offers educational credits and complements oncology workforce development in Africa.

References

[1] Li J 2016 A balanced approach to radiotherapy: integrating cobalt-60 machines and linear accelerators treatment *IAEA News* 28 September www.iaea.org/newscenter/news/a-balanced-approach-to-radiotherapy-integrating-cobalt-60-machines-and-linear-accelerators-treatment

[2] World Health Organization 2011 Procurement process resource guide - WHO Medical device technical series. 2011:38. http://whqlibdoc.who.int/publications/2011/9789241501378_eng.pdf?ua=1 Accessed November 6, 2016.

[3] Our Cancer Prevention Recommendations. World Cancer Research Fund International www.wcrf.org/int/research-we-fund/our-cancer-prevention-recommendations Accessed August 18, 2017

[4] Jemal A, Bray F, Forman D, O'Brien M, Ferlay J, Center M and Parkin D M 2012 Cancer burden in Africa and opportunities for prevention *Cancer* **118** 4372–84

[5] Sitas F, Parkin M, Chirenje Z, Stein L, Mqoqi N and Wabinga H 2006 *Cancers. Disease and Mortality in Sub-Saharan Africa* The International Bank for Reconstruction and Development/The World Bank Retrieved from www.ncbi.nlm.nih.gov/pubmed/21290654

Chapter 7

Quo vadis? Cancer moonshot for global oncology

Eduardo Cazap and Wilfred Ngwa

7.1 The Cancer moonshot

At the American Association of Physicists in Medicine (AAPM) Conference in 2016, the Acting Director of the National Cancer Institute (NCI) provided insights into the Cancer moonshot and other initiatives to accelerate cancer research and make more therapies available to patients. He encouraged the assembled Blue Ribbon Panel of experts made up of cancer researchers, oncologists, patient advocates, and representatives from the private sector and government agencies, to identify scientific opportunities that could be advanced by the Cancer moonshot. They focused on opportunities in seven areas: clinical trials, enhanced data sharing, cancer immunology, implementation science, pediatric cancer, precision prevention and early detection, and tumor evolution and progression. Recommendations made by the panel are listed in table 7.1.

Some of these recommendations are consistent with what the NCI is currently funding with respect to global health. A number of these funding opportunities are highlighted in the lecture by the NCI in chapter 3. During the AAPM conference, the acting director also highlighted several research initiatives on imaging and radiation therapy to better understand how to use immunotherapies in combination with targeted therapies and treatments such as chemotherapy and radiation. While foreign institutions may not apply for this funding, one of the funding opportunity announcements PAR-16-111, allows for foreign components.

Building on this, on 11 January 2017, the NCI launched a new drug formulary (the 'NCI Formulary') that will enable investigators at NCI-designated Cancer Centers to quickly access approved investigational agents for use in preclinical studies and cancer clinical trials. In consonance with the Cancer moonshot initiative goals, the NCI Formulary is a public–private partnership between NCI and pharmaceutical and biotechnology companies, designed to speed-up the availability

doi:10.1088/978-0-7503-1359-9ch7

Table 7.1. Blue Ribbon Panel of experts recommendations for advancing cancer moonshot.

A. Establish a network for direct patient involvement.	Engage patients to contribute their comprehensive tumor profile data to expand knowledge about what therapies work, in whom, and in which types of cancer.
B. Create a translational science network devoted exclusively to immunotherapy.	Establish a cancer immunotherapy network to discover why immunotherapy is effective in some patients but not in others.
C. Develop ways to overcome cancer's resistance to therapy.	Identify therapeutic targets to overcome drug resistance through studies that determine the mechanisms that lead cancer cells to become resistant to previously effective treatments.
D. Build a national cancer data ecosystem.	Create a national ecosystem for sharing and analyzing cancer data so that researchers, clinicians and patients will be able to contribute data, which will facilitate efficient data analysis.
E. Intensify research on the major drivers of childhood cancers.	Improve our understanding of fusion oncoproteins in pediatric cancer and use new preclinical models to develop inhibitors that target them
F. Minimize cancer treatment's debilitating side effects.	Accelerate the development of guidelines for routine monitoring and management of patient-reported symptoms to minimize debilitating side effects of cancer and its treatment.
G. Expand use of proven cancer prevention and early detection strategies.	Reduce cancer risk and cancer health disparities through approaches in development, testing and broad adoption of proven prevention strategies.
H. Mine past patient data to predict future patient outcomes.	Predict response to standard treatments through retrospective analysis of patient specimens.
I. Develop a 3D cancer atlas.	Create dynamic 3D maps of human tumor evolution to document the genetic lesions and cellular interactions of each tumor as it evolves from a precancerous lesion to advanced cancer
J. Develop new cancer technologies.	Develop new enabling cancer technologies to characterize tumors and test therapies

of more-effective treatment options to patients with cancer. It advances the need for greater collaboration and faster development of new therapies or technologies needed for patients. The availability of agents through the NCI Formulary will expedite the start of clinical trials by alleviating the lengthy negotiation process, which sometimes takes up to 18 months, due to the fact that investigators are required to access such agents on their own. The initial NCI Formulary was launched with fifteen targeted agents from six pharmaceutical companies: Bristol-Myers Squibb, Eli Lilly and Company, Genentech, Kyowa Hakko Kirin, Loxo Oncology, and Xcovery Holding Company LLC. Key features emerging from the Cancer moonshot initiative so far are: public–private partnerships, cross-disciplinary collaborations including working with cancer advocates, identified high impact research areas, and the urgency of now, in accelerating research to benefit cancer patients.

7.2 What is the equivalent of the Cancer moonshot for global health?

The Cancer moonshot does not specifically mention global health or efforts beyond the USA. However, if successful, the scientific advances would greatly benefit global health. For example, any new treatments or technologies developed (table 7.1) could also benefit cancer patients in low and middle income countries (LMICs). From the perspective of global health the issues faced by patients in America including disparities, e.g. in clinical trials, are in many ways similar to those faced on a global scale. According to the NCI, the Cancer moonshot to accelerate cancer research aims to make more therapies available to more patients, while also improving our ability to prevent cancer and detect it at an early stage. Its goal is to make a decade worth of progress in five years. For global health, a similar goal would apply, to accelerate efforts to provide more patients with access to cancer prevention and control. Discussions at the yearly Global Health Catalyst (GHC) summit have allowed identifications of specific global oncology areas of focus. Some of these build on the Lancet Oncology Commission report. Some of these goals and the approach to achieve them resonate with those of the NCI Cancer moonshot Blue Ribbon panel. The areas include catalyzing:

1. Public–private partnerships with stakeholders similar to what is being done in the Moonshot initiative, to support the establishment of at least one cancer center with radiotherapy service in each African country by 2022.
2. The establishment of a Virtual Harambee platform which integrates:
    a. ICT-powered global oncology research: the Global Cancer Project Map, with seed-funding for co-mentored research collaborations involving LMIC and high income country faculty and research associates, as well as the establishment of an International Imaging and Radiation Oncology Core (I^2ROC) for the African region building on the NCI-funded QARC, which will facilitate research like multi-center clinical trials.
    b. ICT-powered global oncology education/training: with online education in partnership with the African Organization for Research and Training in Cancer.
    c. ICT-powered global oncology care: integrating a telemedicine platform, eCARE4Africa.
3. The implementation of the 'best buys' for cancer prevention and advocacy highlighted by the lecture of Seun Adebiyi from the American Cancer Society.
4. The implementation of unprecedented collaborations/partnerships with the resource-laden diaspora, athletes, and religious institutions.
5. Continuous knowledge sharing and partnership/collaboration building through the yearly GHC summits.

The first focus area on building public–private partnerships was well addressed by a number of global health leaders at the summit including Doyin Oluwole (Director of the Pink Ribbon Red Ribbon, at President George W Bush Institute) and Eduardo Cazap. The follow section provides lecture notes from Dr Cazap.

7.3 The value of public–private partnerships

Lecture by Professor Eduardo Cazap (Immediate Past President of the Union for International Cancer Control (UICC) and Past President, Latin American & Caribbean Society of Medical Oncology).

7.3.1 Introduction

Currently, millions of people are dying from potentially treatable cancers, such as breast and prostate, because of a chronic underinvestment in radiotherapy resources. New estimates reveal that 204 million fractions of radiotherapy will be needed to treat the 12 million cancer patients worldwide who could benefit from treatment by 2035. Despite the enormity of the problem, the cost per fraction is highly cost-effective and very low compared to the high price of many new cancer drugs. Tackling the global shortfall in radiotherapy could save millions of lives and boost the economy of poorer countries. Investment in radiotherapy services could bring economic benefits of up to US$365 billion in developing countries over the next 20 years. We all know the current situation and the incoming world crisis (the current estimated lack of 7000 radiotherapy centers worldwide). As with the Cancer moonshot's urgency of now, we need urgent solutions applicable to real world situations. Successful examples in LMIC settings could be extrapolated to other world regions (which is a goal of the Harvard Global Catalyst (GCH) Summits in promoting knowledge sharing). One example worth sharing illustrates the value of public–private partnerships (PPPs).

7.3.2 The value of PPP

Several countries and groups are working following this concept. This involves the development of consortia constituted by academic international cooperation, local leaders and institutions, and ministers of health, together with private groups as useful partners. A true cooperation in cases where each stakeholder alone is unable to develop the project shows better outcomes. A good example is the Rwanda case. This project is based on the PPP concept, extrapolation of successful experiences in similar contexts, implementation of real world actions, and cost-effectiveness of radiotherapy. The partners included: Partners In Health (PIH)/Inshuti Mu Buzima Rwanda, Global Health Equity@ Harvard Medical School, Latin-American & Caribbean Society of Medical Oncology (SLACOM), Center for Global Cancer Medicine, Abramson Cancer Center, University of Pennsylvania, USA, Rwanda Military Hospital, Kigali and Butaro Hospital, Butaro, Rwanda, Rwanda Minister of Health (MOH), and 21st Century Oncology. Some leaders in this effort included: Dr Triedman, a radiation oncologist at Brown University who has been consulting with PIH and the Rwandan MOH on the development radiation plans in Rwanda;

Professor Ahmed Elzawawy, an extraordinary facilitator in global actions; Lawrence N Shulman, Director, Center for Global Cancer Medicine, Abramson Cancer Center, University of Pennsylvania; Dr Park, the Director of NCDs with Partners in Health (PIH) that oversees oncology care at Butaro hospital and works closely with the MOH of Rwanda. In this PPP, 21st Century Oncology was an important partner (figure 7.1). This physician-led provider has already successfully realized PPP projects in Las Vegas (Nevada), Jacksonville (Florida), Irazu (Costa Rica), San Juan (Argentina), and Hospital Austral (Argentina).

In one case in Santo Domingo, Dominican Republic, a new state-of-the-art cancer center was constructed on the hospital's campus with a signed long-term lease contract purchasing a new Varian linear accelerator (LINAC). A loan was provided for this project by the International Finance Corporation (World Bank Group). The center successfully opened in 2014. The market view was such that a third of the country's residents live in the relevant geographic area. The hospital partnered with 21st Century Oncology to promote the center outside the Dominican Republic

In another case in Tijuana Mexico, a cancer center was identified which was using 25+ year-old technology. The previous owners elected to sell instead of making costly investments in the center leasehold improvements and modern equipment. The center was rented from the prior owners under a long-term agreement. The center was refurbished, brought up to code, installed with a Varian LINAC and opened in May 2015. This is an underseved market of 4 million people with one

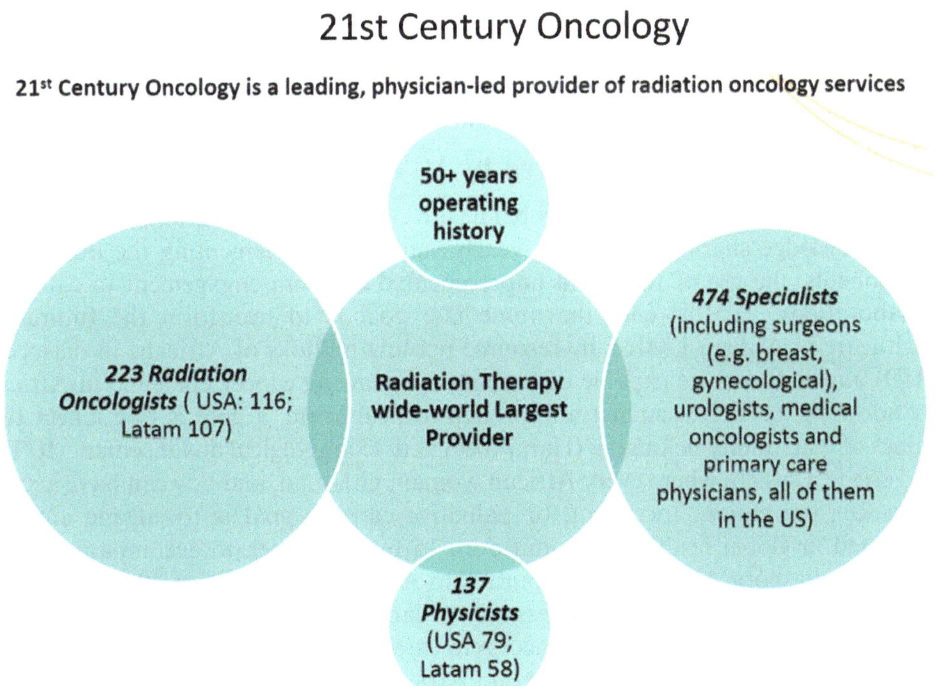

Figure 7.1. 21st century oncology.

competitor who is using a cobalt-60 machine. International Finance Corporation also provided a loan for the project. Mexican regulators are increasingly strict, less willing to renew cobalt licenses, essentially encouraging technology transition. However, cobalt to LINAC involves constructing a new vault, leasehold improvements, and machine replacement.

A final case is in Santiago, Dominican Republic, involving a public hospital with 50 years of operation, which needed to discontinue use of a cobalt machine. The public hospital did not have capital to modernize. A new vault was built to install a modern Varian LINAC. In the hospital arrangement, a long-term lease contract was finalized in 2015 with plans to install the LINAC in 2016. One partner was to operate the center and pay the hospital rent. The partnership benefits included: elevating quality of care available to public hospital patients, access to a premier global radiation oncology network, and an offer to local partners/physicians with an option to purchase membership interest. In the market view, this is the second largest city in the country with two other competitors with LINACs.

The take-home messages in all of these examples are that the implementation, development, installation, training, and maintenance of low cost, good quality radiation services in LMICs is feasible. This innovative PPP strategy could be tested in Africa. Multisectoral consortiums and partnerships with proven experience are critical to achieve success. If the Rwanda case is accomplished it may be followed by other institutions, cities. and countries

Another area or approach adopted by the Harvard GHC is the use of advanced information and communication technologies (ICTs) to catalyze collaborations that will accelerate global oncology benefits for cancer patients. This is captured by the GHC's virtual Harambee platform.

7.4 Virtual Harambee powered by ICTs and the diaspora

The GHC's model for catalyzing global health collaborations leverages three things, with knowledge sharing during the yearly summits complementing the other two components: the use of ICTs and unprecedented diaspora engagement to catalyze collaborations. To this end, the immediate goal is to transform the future of healthcare in African LMICs by resource pooling millions of Africans in diaspora (AiD) and well-wishers capable of curbing the growing cancer epidemic in Africa. By adopting an interdisciplinary approach to healthcare, a goal is to connect the values of community belonging (Harambee) with technological advancement (ICTs) and create a system where every African woman, girl, man, and boy can have access to cancer prevention, treatment, or palliative care. A goal is to engage anyone interested in global health to commit even 15 min per week to accompany others including diaspora Africans, on a journey to Africa, where at least 300 000 people can be prevented from dying unnecessarily of cancer per year, just because they were born there, and so have little or no access to care. The model could then be extended in the long term to other LMICs beyond Africa. The virtual Harambee platform is designed to catalyze international collaborations in global oncology research, education, and care.

Going forward, in research, the virtual Harambee will integrate ICT-powered global oncology research: the Global Cancer Project Map, with seed-funding for co-mentored research collaborations involving LMIC and high income country faculty and research associates. This program was pioneered at the 2017 GHC summit with seed funding provided by crowd-funding by diaspora organizations. Also in research the virtual Harambee platform will integrate an International Imaging and Radiation Oncology Core (I^2ROC) for the African region, building on the NCI-funded QARC, which will facilitate research including multi-center clinical trials, which are one of the key sessions of the summits going forward.

Meanwhile, in education/training, the Harambee platform will integrate online education in partnership with the African Organization for Research and Training in Cancer. The 2017 certificate courses include: mixed methods research, clinical trials, psycho-oncology, molecular pathology, basic and translational research, medical oncology, advocacy, and global radiation oncology. The global radiation oncology course will cover high impact topics, such as radiation safety, treatment planning, and quality assurance, and innovative areas such as nanomedicine, genetics, and so forth, which can be supported remotely, as described in previous publications [1].

Finally, the virtual Harambee platform will support a telemedicine platform, eCARE4Africa, that will allow for cancer care professionals anywhere in the world, including from the diaspora, to pool their time together to support local doctors in Africa to provide greater access to cancer care, including providing a second opinion. In this model, some local health professionals in Africa may play a main role of reviewing and signing off on input from outside Africa. Details and progress evaluation will be made during the yearly GHC summits.

7.5 Other focus areas on the global oncology moonshot emerging from the Harvard GHC summits

Other focus areas emerging from the yearly GHC summits include a focus on the 'best buys' in cancer prevention and advocacy. These best buys, highlighted by the lecture from the American Cancer Society in chapter 5, include HPV screening and curbing the use of tobacco by advocating for higher taxes, as shown by the successful case of Brazil. Going forward there will also be greater focus on the implementation of unprecedented collaborations/partnerships with athletes, and religious institutions and the resource-laden diaspora.

The initial focus on Africa is due to the fact that it arguably has the greatest need at present for collaborations in global oncology. Currently the second most populated and the fastest growing continent, Africa represents a youthful energetic space that will dramatically shape the future of the world. Many studies and publications show that the African diaspora has a significant sphere of cultural, financial, and spiritual influence on Africa as their ancestral or adoptive home. This influence is bolstered by over $50 billion dollars in remittances per year, which is more than foreign aid to the continent. The resource-laden AiD is considered to be a third of Africa's brain power and the African Union now officially recognizes the new African diaspora as the sixth sub-region of Africa. Surveys show over 90% of these new diasporans want to participate in collective efforts to transform their sending continent, invest in Africa's health, and therefore in Africa's future. The virtual Harambee is designed to turn the brain drain to a major gain in healthcare.

Key elements for preventing the cancer epidemic in Africa already exist, including the intellectual force from a passionate African diaspora and so many good-willed non-Africans, low-cost technologies, a growing upsurge in global health interest, and clinical expertise necessary to reduce the burden of human illness. What has been missing is a systematic and creative way to make otherwise dispersed professional competence due to brain drain available to those in need. The GHC's virtual Harambee infrastructure provides just such a platform; it integrates interdisciplinary competencies in the scientific, technological, and social sciences to make it easy for people anywhere to participate and curb the growing cancer epidemic in LMICs, make an impact in communal health, and save lives. In this volume we have documented stories of how the AiD is enhancing access to cancer prevention, treatment, and palliative care in partnership with hundreds of AiD groups and well-wishers.

Quite importantly, anyone can be involved in this vision of where the virtual Harambee could take us. Simply log-on to the Harambee platform from your computer, pick your country of choice, and spend 15 min making a potentially life-saving impact, while learning something about the local culture or country in the process. You can enter your expertise and the Harambee platform will tell you how you can help: creating cancer awareness; participating in education, e.g. educate a women's group about cancer (most of Africa's over 2000 languages do not have a word for cancer); e-advocate on behalf of those socially ostracized because of their illnesses; give a second opinion or consult a patient; e-hug or pray with a cancer patient; e-teach, e-research/mentor a student's research project; collaborate with faculty or health-professionals; participate in an innovation hub or venture accelerator on low cost healthcare tech for which you can invest in, etc. At the end of each month, you get feedback on your Harambee impact or tax-deductible time and efforts to reverse cancer trends in Africa. Beyond individual participation, institutions—churches, hospitals, diaspora groups, NGOs, etc—can participate and leave a collective impact, transforming communities and saving lives. The sustainable approach could subsequently be scaled/adapted to other diseases or regions of the world.

Finally, going forward, a focus will continue to be on knowledge sharing and partnership/collaboration building through the yearly GHC summits. Outcomes will include: yearly publications and dissemination of the conference proceedings; live online courses from Harvard Medical School each year; providing crowdfunding support by the diaspora to seed co-mentored research collaborations across the Atlantic; awards and networking with global health leaders and stakeholders; new partnerships to develop or support cancer centers in African countries; telemedicine; mobilization of hundreds of Africans in diaspora groups united against cancer; multi-center clinical trials initiatives with LMIC cancer centers; and more partnerships to catalyze high impact international collaborations to save lives and eliminate cancer disparities. All of this boils down to catalyzing global oncology collaborations geared towards accelerating access to cancer care for patients in LMICs *until every patient has access to cancer prevention, treatment, or palliative care*. This is the evident global oncology moonshot emerging from the Harvard GHC summits: accelerating collaborations to realize the dream that one day cancer will be eradicated, and that people of all socio-economic, racial, religious, and cultural backgrounds will have access to quality healthcare.

Reference

[1] Ngwa W and Ngoma T 2016 *Emerging Models for Global Health in Radiation Oncology* (Bristol: IOP Publishing)

Lightning Source UK Ltd.
Milton Keynes UK
UKOW07n1426190917
309478UK00003B/41/P

9 780750 313605